About the author

Marilyn Glenville PhD is the UK's leading expert in nutritional health for women. She obtained her doctorate from Cambridge University and is a Fellow of the Royal Society of Medicine and a member of the Nutrition Society.

For over 25 years Dr Glenville has studied and practised nutrition, both in the UK and in the US. She has had several papers published in scientific journals, frequently advises health professionals and often lectures at academic conferences held at the Medical Society, the Royal College of Physicians and the Royal College of Surgeons. She is also a popular international speaker. As a respected author on women's healthcare she gives regular talks on radio and has often appeared on television and in the press.

Dr Glenville is the President of the Food and Health Forum at the Royal Society of Medicine, patron of the Daisy Network (a charity for premature menopause) and a member of the British Fertility Society. She was formerly an observer on the Foods Standards Agency's Expert Group on the safety of vitamins and minerals, and is also a Fellow of the Royal Society of Arts.

Dr Glenville is the author of eight internationally best-selling books on health: *Fat Around the Middle, The New Natural Alternatives to HRT, Healthy Eating for the Menopause, Natural Solutions to Infertility, The Nutritional Health Handbook for Women, Overcoming PMS the Natural Way* and *Osteoporosis – The Silent Epidemic.*

Dr Glenville runs her own clinics in London and Tunbridge Wells (see page 224 for details) and also has a non-commercial website: *www.marilynglenville.com*

'Marilyn Glenville is one of the UK's foremost nutritionists and she and I have worked together since 1995. We practise integrated healthcare where nutrition is combined with medical treatment to help families with fertility issues. The results have been astounding and I am sure that this integrated approach is the way forward in patient care. Marilyn's books are always easy to read, informative and very practical. This book is no exception.' *Mr Yehudi Gordon MB, Bch, MD, FRCOG, Consultant gynaecologist and obstetrician*

Dr Gordon is one of the UK's most sought-after gynaecologists and the founder of Viveka – clinic for integrated health. He has pioneered the integrated approach to the diagnosis and treatment of fertility difficulties, pelvic pain and menstrual disorders. He is also an advocate of active and water birth and has changed the face of obstetrics in the UK: he set up the birth unit at the Hospital of St John and St Elizabeth where he also works as a consultant obstetrician.

'Working in a multi-disciplinary team that includes complementary and medical professionals greatly enhances the effect on couples seeking fertility treatment. Working with Dr Glenville, closely developing paths for couples to improve their fertility and general health before embarking on a pregnancy, has been a major factor in Viveka's success. Marilyn's expertise, highly up-to-date ideas, innovation on how to improve the health of couples through lifestyle, nutrition and supplements make a real impact on achieving a successful pregnancy and healthy child.' *Mr Talha Shawaf MB, ChB, FRSC(Ed), FRCOG, Consultant at Bart's and the London Centre for Reproductive Medicine NHS Trust*

His interest in fertility began over 20 years ago, during which time he has built up a profound experience in all aspects of infertility management and has written over 60 articles and chapters in books.

'Within the medical profession we are becoming increasingly aware of the benefits of expert nutritional advice in the management of a wide variety of diseases. Most subfertility is not associated with an obvious pathological process, but the delicate eggs and sperm need an optimum environment in order to thrive. We are delighted to work closely with Dr Glenville who provides expert scientific advice in this area whilst we concentrate on the more clinical treatments. This complementary, holistic approach has undoubted benefits for our patients.' *Mr Mark Wilcox, DM FRCOG, Fertility Specialist, South East Fertility Clinic*

From the parents

'I originally came to see you with my husband for advice on how to get my periods back to being regular. I have since found out that I am pregnant, which is fantastic.'

'He's been an absolute joy since he arrived and seems to be progressing frighteningly fast, smiling at anyone who cares to pay him attention and already holding his head up unsupported. The midwives marvelled at how healthy he was and I heard one say I obviously had a very healthy diet – again thanks to you!'

'She was conceived naturally after two failed IVF cycles – thank you so much for your help … all is going well, she is wonderful and we couldn't be happier.'

'Many thanks for all your help and support during our IVF treatment. Our son is just perfect. Your nutritional advice made such a difference not just in terms of preparing us for IVF but also for our health generally. We are now lifelong converts to your healthy eating approach.'

'I am the lady with high FSH (50+, age 41) who had a baby following your diet, after being told I had a less than 1 per cent chance of conceiving. My husband and I want to pass on our heartfelt thanks to you for helping to bring our baby son into the world. We really cannot thank you enough for the tremendous difference you have made to our lives in helping this 'high FSH' lady have a baby, so long hoped for.'

'At last I have the opportunity to send you a photo of our little miracle. She is of course very precious, even if she does keep us up most nights! Thank you for your help and support over the last couple of years, which as you know, were very difficult times.'

'Who said there's no life in the old dog yet, 44+!'

'The advice for me was critical, as no-one else offered it (and I looked everywhere) – Marilyn is wonderful!'

Getting pregnant *faster*

Boost your
fertility in just
3 months

Dr Marilyn Glenville PhD

Kyle Cathie Ltd

First published in Great Britain in 2008 by
Kyle Cathie Limited
122 Arlington Road, London NW1 7HP
general.enquiries@kyle-cathie.com
www.kylecathie.com

10 9 8 7 6 5 4 3 2 1

ISBN 978-1-85626-760-1

Project editor: Jennifer Wheatley
Designer: Jane Humphrey
Illustrations: John Erwood
Copy editor: Anne Newman
Editorial assistant: Vicki Murrell
Production: Sha Huxtable

A Cataloguing In Publication record for this title is
available from the British Library.

Printed and bound by Martins the Printers Ltd,
Berwick upon Tweed

Disclaimer The contents of this book are for information
only and are intended to assist readers in identifying
symptoms and conditions they may be experiencing. This
book is not intended to be a substitute for taking proper
medical advice and should not be relied upon in this way.
Always consult a qualified doctor or health practitioner.
The author and publisher cannot accept responsibility for
illness arising out of the failure to seek medical advice
from a doctor.

To my happy, healthy granddaughter,
Katie Sophia Glenville
(born in August 2006),
with love from Nana

Acknowledgements

This book has been a pleasure to write because it will give many couples the information they need to have the baby they long for. There is nothing more fulfilling than to receive a letter or a photograph from a couple who never thought they would have a baby.

I would like to thank Theresa Cheung for all the help she gave me in making the writing as easy as possible. My thanks also go to Jenny Wheatley, my editor at Kyle Cathie, and Anne Newman, my copy editor, who had the task of whittling the word count down as I seemed to have so much to say. I would like to say a big thank you to Kyle herself, who I have worked with now for ten years and it is a pleasure to work with her each time.

It is a pleasure and privilege to work with fertility specialists who have such an interest and open-mindedness for the nutritional approach to fertility and use it alongside the conventional investigations and treatments. It gives couples such confidence that they are being looked after holistically and that everybody is communicating with each other in what is the best treatment plan for each couple. I would especially like to thank Yehudi Gordon, consultant gynaecologist and obstetrician, who has been a pioneer in this integrated approach to health and who founded Viveka healthcare centre in London, and Talha Shawaf, reproductive medicine specialist, who has such a vast reservoir of knowledge on the evidence-based approaches to fertility. Thanks also to Michael Rimington and Mark Wilcox of the South East Fertility Clinic in Tunbridge Wells who are such forward thinkers in this area of fertility.

As with my other books, it would not be possible to have the time to write without the support of the team at the Tunbridge Wells clinic. My special thanks go to Mel, Helen, Brenda, Sharon, Gayla, Katie, Lisa, Len, Nick and Lee who are so supportive.

My love also goes to my family: Kriss, my husband, and my three children Matt, Len and Chantell.

introduction

FERTILITY FACTS AND HOW TO GET THE BEST FROM THIS BOOK

This book has been designed for you as an individual. No two couples are ever alike in terms of what may be preventing them from getting pregnant, which is why it is so important to have all the information that addresses your needs – which can be very different from those of another couple – at your fingertips. From many years' experience of helping couples to become parents it is clear that a well-structured plan is needed – one that ticks all the boxes – so that you know what you should be doing and when, in order not to waste time.

This book is for any woman who wants to have a baby, from those who are thinking about it for the first time to those who have been trying for months or years without results. You can also use it if you are going for IVF, IUI or ICSI as it will prepare your body for that treatment cycle, giving you the best chance of success. Couples who have already had a baby will find the book useful if they are struggling to conceive again (secondary infertility) as all the recommendations can help you to get pregnant faster. It will also be beneficial to those who are going for egg or sperm donation and those who have had one or more miscarriage.

The book shows you how an integrated approach to getting and staying pregnant gives you the best of both worlds through a combination of conventional and nutritional medicine. It is important to know that you are taking all the right steps and in the right order and this book takes you logically through those steps, just as if you were having a consultation at one of my clinics (see page 224 for more information). The aim is the same as the clinics' – to find out what is preventing you from getting or staying pregnant. If we can find the cause we can treat it. It may be a nutritional or lifestyle issue and making changes in those areas will be enough; or it may be a combination of medical and nutritional factors in which case all of those need to be addressed and corrected.

If you and your partner are having problems conceiving, doing everything you can to boost your fertility is important. It could well make the difference between you being able to conceive easily and then carrying a healthy baby to full term – or not.

using this book

BASIC FERTILITY FACTS

The usual statistic[1] quoted for couples seeking medical help for infertility is one in seven but a UK National Fertility Survey, published in September 2007, suggests that fertility problems are more than twice as common as previously thought, with up to a third of couples struggling to conceive, many of them not seeking help or advice. This means that as many as one in three of us could at some stage in our lives be going through the anxiety and stress – often in secret – of wondering whether we'll ever have a child. Some of that anxiety and stress could be eased if we knew some basic fertility facts[2] and exactly what we could do to increase our chances of having a healthy baby.

DON'T ASSUME IT WILL HAPPEN RIGHT AWAY!

As women, we spend most of our reproductive life trying not to get pregnant and then to find out that getting pregnant isn't as easy for you as it seems to be for others can feel absolutely awful.

A healthy couple at prime reproductive age (below 35) has about a 25 per cent chance of conceiving each month. Only about half of all couples get pregnant within six months of trying, about 80 per cent within a year and approximately 90 per cent at the end of two years. This means that, even if there is nothing wrong with you, it can take you up to eighteen months, even two years to conceive. Over the age of 30, it may take even longer. So how do you know when something's amiss?

The answer can depend on age.[3] Women under the age of 35 are advised to seek treatment for infertility if they haven't become pregnant after 12 months of regular unprotected sex. For those over 35, the threshold is three to six months instead of 12.

Age, however, isn't the only factor. Human fertility is extremely complex[4] and every aspect needs to be taken into account from your diet and lifestyle to your medical history, current stress level and any environmental and occupational hazards. The good news is that many of the factors involved in fertility are within your control and the eight-step fertility-boosting programme in this book will show you all the things you can do to conceive a healthy baby – faster.

YOUR INDIVIDUAL NEEDS

My fertility plan has been designed specifically to resolve whatever factors may be stopping you getting pregnant. The three-month fertility plan will help to make sure that everything that needs to be tested or checked *is* tested and checked and at the right time. It will also introduce you to the very latest research on diet, lifestyle and techniques that can make all the difference. You do not have to read the whole book or plough through topics that are not applicable to you; the guide below will point you in the direction of those sections that are relevant to you.

	If you have been trying to conceive for over six months but not more than 12	If you have been trying to conceive for 12 months or more	If you have had one or more miscarriages
If you are under 35	As you are under the age of 35, you have some time to put into place the plan in Steps 1–5 over the next three months. Then give yourselves six months to conceive naturally, using the information in Step 6 and if it has not happened then, go to Step 7.	As you are under the age of 35, you have some time to put into place the plan in Steps 1–5 over the next three months. Read Step 6 as you try to conceive naturally over the next three months and if it has not happened then go to Step 7.	Follow Steps 1–5 for three months before you try again. Pay particular attention to Step 5 and get any infections checked, treated and re-tested so that you or your partner are clear before you get pregnant again.
If you are over 35	Unfortunately, fertility declines dramatically from the age of 35, so you need to run Steps 1–5 and Step 7 concurrently in order to rule out medical problems. If you get a diagnosis of unexplained infertility then give yourself six months to reap the benefits of Steps 1–5, also putting into place Step 6. Then if you are not pregnant go on to Step 8.	Fertility declines dramatically from the age of 35, so you need to run Steps 1–5 and Step 7 concurrently in order to rule out medical problems. If you get a diagnosis of unexplained infertility then give yourself three months to reap the benefits of Steps 1–5, also putting into place Step 6. Then if you are not pregnant go on to Step 8.	Follow Steps 1–5 for three months, paying particular attention to Step 5 and getting any infections treated and re-tested to get the all clear. At the same time, go to Step 7 and have the tests that are related to miscarriage. It is pointless to embark on IVF if you have not covered all these steps as your problem has not been getting pregnant but staying pregnant. I have seen couples with recurrent miscarriage go on to have IVF and just have another miscarriage because the cause of the miscarriages was not addressed.

PRE-CONCEPTION CARE

Getting pregnant and having a healthy baby isn't just about sex! Research[5] shows that everything you do in the three or four months before trying to conceive can be as important as the sex itself. What you eat, drink, breathe, do as a job, how stressed you are – it all matters not just to your fertility but also to the health of your baby to be.

The egg and sperm released at conception are the products of your own and your partner's diet and lifestyle and researchers now believe that these factors prior to conception are just as significant to the health of your future baby as they are during pregnancy. If you are undernourished there is even the terrifying possibility that your baby could well become 'programmed' at conception to have a higher risk of future health problems, such as high blood pressure, diabetes and obesity. Which is why I always recommend a three-month period of pre-conception care.

Most pre-conception care is straightforward DIY diet and lifestyle measures to get you and your partner as healthy as possible before you try for a baby. Remember, this isn't just to boost fertility, it is also because the healthier you are before you get pregnant or start fertility treatment, the better your chances of having a healthy pregnancy, easier delivery and a healthy baby.

WHY YOUR PARTNER NEEDS TO WORK WITH YOU

A good pre-conception care programme involves getting both you and your partner in the best possible physical and mental shape before you try for a baby. In couples with fertility problems, it is thought that approximately one third could be attributed to the male partner, one third to the female partner and one third to a combination of both.

For men, the most common problem is not just the quantity but the quality of sperm – are they strong, normal and fit enough to reach and penetrate a ripe egg? Sperm quality and quantity can be affected by lifestyle factors such as poor diet, stress, smoking and alcohol, which means that men have a great deal of control over their own fertility. Indeed, studies[6] show that simple changes (as recommended in Steps 1 to 4 of this book), can improve sperm quantity and quality in as little as three months.

Working to improve your health and fertility together is important. Although you are the one who is going to be pregnant, never lose sight of the fact that getting pregnant takes two.

WHY THREE MONTHS?

The eight-step fertility-boosting programme is designed for a period of at least three months. This is the recommended period of time for pre-conception care because it takes approximately that long for the follicles on your ovaries to develop before one is mature enough to release an egg at ovulation. Approximately 20 follicles, all containing the developing eggs, grow on the ovary surface in each menstrual cycle. In most cases, however, it is just the largest follicle that continues to develop, and this is why most couples only have one baby. The others degenerate and are re-absorbed. Sometimes two eggs are released from two separate follicles in one cycle and non-identical twins would be conceived.

Most women are born with about 2 million egg follicles; by puberty there are about 750,000, and by the age of around 45, as few as 10,000 may be left. So although you cannot change the number of eggs you have, you can change their quality and this is the crucial point. By improving the quality of your eggs, you are increasing your chances of conceiving naturally and also preventing a miscarriage. If you are going for an assisted conception technique, like IUI, IVF or ICSI, you will also want your eggs to be as healthy as possible so as to give the technique the best chance. With a national average success rate for IVF of just 25 per cent, it is important to do whatever you can.

With men, it also takes at least three months for a new batch of sperm cells to mature, ready to be ejaculated. Men produce sperm all their lives so it is always possible not only to improve the quality but also the quantity with lifestyle and nutritional changes.

In addition, it can take from six weeks to three months to eliminate certain toxins from your system properly, and to raise the level of crucial fertility-boosting nutrients in your bloodstream. Research spearheaded by European doctors suggests that a good three-month programme of healthy living and eating will maximise your chances of conception, whether you want to try now or in the future.[7]

Finally, three months is the recommended period of time for dietary changes to take effect and for nutritional and herbal supplements to work their magic. And according to psychologists it also takes at least three months to replace dietary and lifestyle habits with healthier ones. Think about it – old habits die hard and your body and mind need that period to adjust to fertility and health-boosting changes.[8]

PUTTING YOU IN CONTROL

My aim in writing this book is to put *you* in the driving seat. I strongly advise you to incorporate as many of my recommendations into your diet and lifestyle as possible. Then, knowing that you are doing absolutely everything you can to boost your fertility will give you the peace of mind you need to get on with the rest of your life and, more important than you think, to enjoy baby-making.

The eight-step plan that follows has helped many of my patients to become pregnant, cut their risk of miscarriage and have healthy babies. It can help you too.

step one
your diet

....

If you're sceptical about the connection between food and fertility bear in mind that your body uses the nutrients from the food that you eat – and the supplements that you take – to repair cells, produce hormones and ultimately produce healthy eggs and sperm. In many ways your fertility depends upon what you eat.

A healthy, nutrient-rich, balanced diet in the pre-conception period will not only boost your chances of getting pregnant and having a healthy baby, it will also keep your blood sugar levels in balance and your weight under control. As you'll see in more detail later in this chapter, if your blood sugar is not balanced, or if you are under- or overweight, the reproductive hormones which control your fertility will not work properly, severely limiting your chances of conceiving. Many of the women I treat in my clinic who are having problems getting pregnant exhibit at least one or more major nutritional deficiency and have chaotic blood sugar levels. A healthy, well-balanced diet of fresh, whole foods is therefore the cornerstone of my fertility-boosting action plan.

Standard medical advice is to get all the nutrients you need from a good balanced diet. Unfortunately, even if you do try to eat healthily the food you eat may not always contain all that you need. It has become apparent that women are not even getting enough of the most basic nutrient for pregnancy, folic acid. The National Diet and Nutrition Survey[1] showed that a staggering 84 per cent of women fail to achieve the Reference Nutrient Intake (RNI – this replaced the Recommended Daily Allowance or RDA) for folic acid leading to the proposal that bread should be fortified with this vitamin. Overall, 74 per cent of women are falling short on nutrients from their diet, with an 80 per cent decrease in the consumption of omega 3 fatty acids[2] and an intake of 50 per cent more saturated fat than the maximum recommended. In general, even with all the government messages, only 15 per cent of women and 13 per cent of men actually meet the five-a-day target for fruit and vegetables.

There is no getting away from the fact that the manufacturing and processing of food today strips essential fertility-boosting nutrients, like zinc, from food. In fact, according to joint research by the Royal Society of Chemistry and the Ministry of

Agriculture and Food, the vitamin and mineral content of fresh foods we buy has been dropping steadily since the 1940s.[3]

With the dominance of supermarket shopping, there's no real way of knowing the freshness or nutritional content of food. A Consumer *Which?* Report in June 2004 found, for example, that packs of sliced green beans contained only 11 per cent of the vitamin C they should have. Other studies have shown significant mineral depletion across a wide range of meat and dairy foods, compared with figures from the 1930s.

This is why on top of a healthy diet plan I also recommend a fertility-boosting supplement plan in Step 3. Supplements (as the name suggests) are no substitute for a healthy diet, as your body digests and absorbs nutrients far better from food than from pills, but they are certainly a good insurance policy.

WHAT IS A FERTILITY-BOOSTING DIET?

In short, it is one that includes all the essential nutrients for conception and pregnancy as well as helping you to balance your blood sugar levels and maintain healthy digestion and the correct weight.

Bear in mind that although I use the term 'diet' in this chapter I do not mean a weight-loss or fad diet – I don't recommend dieting in that sense or excluding food groups while trying for a baby.

Good nutrition does not mean having to give up all the foods you like; it simply means eating more of the right foods and cutting back on the others. Moderation is the key; it's fine to allow yourself the occasional indulgence as long as you are eating healthily at least 80 per cent of the time. And you'll notice that if food cravings have been a problem for you in the past, they will disappear quickly because your body is getting all the nutrients it needs from food that is completely satisfying – so you don't ever feel hungry.

YOUR PRE-CONCEPTION FERTILITY-BOOSTING DIET

Your aim is to ensure you include all the vital food groups – sufficient intake of carbohydrates, fibre and essential fats, healthy amounts of protein and lots of water – in your diet three months before you start trying for a baby. Try to incorporate into your diet as many of the guidelines below as you can.

WATER

Water is an essential but often forgotten ingredient in a healthy eating plan. Not only is your body two thirds water but water intake and distribution are essential for hormonal balance. Water also provides the means for nutrients to travel to all your organs, including your reproductive organs and for toxins to be removed. In addition it helps your body to metabolise stored fat so it is crucial for weight management.

Try to drink at least 1½ litres (or six to eight glasses) of water a day – more if you are also drinking tea and coffee. You should also drink more if you are active, travelling by plane or if you are near central heating. This may seem a lot but after a few days you will soon get used to it.

Generally speaking, mineral water is best. Tap water can be contaminated with heavy metals and other impurities, and some studies have suggested a link between tap water and an increased risk of miscarriage. But don't panic – tap water is the next best choice to mineral water as long as you filter it.[4] Water filters are easily available and the sooner you get into the habit of filtering before you drink or use the water for cooking or making hot drinks the better. If you aren't sure if you are drinking enough keep a record for a few days.

Don't save all your water for mealtimes; drinking while you eat can dilute important digestive enzymes that help break down food. And make sure you drink the right kind of drinks such as diluted fruit juices, smoothies, herbal teas and, of course, water. Tea, coffee, caffeinated and soft fizzy drinks (not sparkling mineral water, this is all right but may make you gassy) don't count because they have a diuretic effect, unsettle your blood sugar levels and don't hydrate your body sufficiently. Drink fluids at room temperature. Cold drinks can shock the body.

IDEAS FOR INCLUDING MORE FLUIDS IN YOUR DIET
~ Keep a jug of water close to you at all times, to remind you to drink regularly. Or you could carry a water bottle with you.
~ Add some lemon if you get bored with plain water.
~ Experiment with herbal teas. Good ones to try are peppermint, chamomile and fennel.
~ Try watered-down fruit juices or diluted fresh pressed juice.
~ Experiment with fruit and vegetables (they are 90 per cent water) in smoothies and soups.

CARBOHYDRATES

Carbohydrates are your key energy source. There are two types – complex and simple. Complex include vegetables and whole grains, such as rye and wheat, and legumes, such as peas and beans. Simple include white sugar, fruit and fruit juices.

For optimum fertility you should limit your intake of simple carbohydrates (with the exception of fruit) and eat plenty of unrefined complex carbohydrates. This means choosing whole-grain bread, brown rice, whole-grain cereals and pasta instead of the refined white versions, and at least five portions of vegetables each day. Whole grains are packed with fertility-boosting nutrients, such as zinc, selenium and many B vitamins, and they are an essential part of a hormone-balancing, fertility-boosting diet.[5]

Steer clear of white flour and other refined grains which have little or no nutritional value because of the processing. In order to digest and absorb refined foods your body has to use its own vitamins and minerals, thus depleting your stores. Simple carbohydrates in the form of sweets, cakes, pies, pastry, white flour, white sugar and refined foods all produce a sudden rise in blood sugar and trigger hormonal imbalances so it is important to avoid them. Fruits are the exception here as although they are simple carbohydrates they are packed with fertility-boosting nutrients. You shouldn't cut fruit out but make sure you eat it with proteins, such as a few nuts or seeds, or some organic live plain yogurt, which can slow down the effect on blood sugar. Make sure too that fruit juices are diluted.

CARBOHYDRATE SPOT CHECK *Include:* whole grains, oats, wholemeal pasta, rye, corn, millet, wholemeal bread, brown rice, buckwheat, raw vegetables, steamed vegetables, fresh fruit, beans and pulses (kidney beans, chick peas, adzuki beans, lentils) *Avoid:* sugar, white flour, white bread, white pasta, biscuits, sweets, puddings, soft fizzy drinks, undiluted fruit juice.

FIVE A DAY Eating five portions of fruit and vegetables a day ensures you get good levels of fertility-boosting antioxidant nutrients like vitamins C and E. Studies have shown that vitamin C has a significant impact on both sperm motility and conception and a sufficient intake of all of these vitamins is of real importance for the production of healthy eggs and sperm. According to a recent study, eating fruit and vegetables daily could potentially halve the risk of miscarriage. A study of thousands of pregnant women revealed that those who had included fruit and vegetables regularly in their diet were 46 per cent less likely to miscarry.[6]

FIBRE

Whole grains, fruits and vegetables provide you with plenty of fibre needed to keep your bowels healthy. It is also vital for fertility because it helps to keep the reproductive system in optimum condition by clearing out toxins and old hormone residues and ensuring that good nutrition gets in. It isn't difficult to increase your fibre intake. You don't need to add bran to everything (bran can actually block the absorption of vital nutrients such as iron and zinc) – just eat more complex carbohydrates: whole-grain rice, oats and bread, and plenty of fruits, vegetables, beans, nuts and seeds.

If you suffer from constipation one tablespoon of whole organic linseeds soaked overnight in water and swallowed in the morning can help to soften stools. Eat a mixture of soluble fibre, such as fruit, oats, vegetables and beans and insoluble (which doesn't dissolve in water), found in whole grains and nuts. Meals loaded with vegetables, cereals, whole grains, nuts and seeds should provide all the fibre you need.

PROTEIN

Protein is important for your fertility because it helps to maintain blood sugar balance and gives your body the even supply of amino acids it needs for building and repairing cells, manufacturing hormones and a healthy reproductive function. Since your body can't store protein the way it does carbohydrate and fat, you need a constant supply and should aim to eat some high-quality protein with every meal.

Different protein sources vary in the amount of other nutrients they contain, so it's important to eat a wide variety. Good sources of protein include oily fish, eggs, pulses, beans, nuts and seeds. Try to have a handful of nuts and seeds every day or use a salad dressing made with a good-quality nut or seed oil. Instead of meat, eat pulses such as lentils, nuts and seeds like sunflower, sesame and quinoa (cooks like a grain but is actually a seed), which are good sources of fertility-boosting protein. New research shows that eating an egg for breakfast not only gives you a protein boost but also keeps you feeling fuller for longer. Up to five eggs a week is perfectly safe for most people. Choose organic, free range eggs because the chicken's diet is extremely important to the quality of the eggs.[7]

Red meat consumption has been linked to fibroids and endometriosis, both of which are oestrogen-dependent conditions that can affect fertility. We also know that more than one and a half servings (125g) of red meat a week can double the risk of breast cancer compared with 0.75 servings a week.[8]

The saturated fats in red meat and poultry produce inflammatory prostaglandins – hormone-like substances which can trigger symptoms of endometriosis, a major cause of fertility problems. According to one study,[9] women following a high animal-protein diet were more likely to have problems conceiving and less likely to carry a pregnancy to full term. High intake of beef, red meat and ham increased the risk of endometriosis by 80 per cent, whereas women with the highest intake of fresh fruit and vegetables lowered their risk by about 40 per cent.

And, according to the very latest research[10], there is also a link between red meat consumption and an increased risk of breast cancer. Carcinogenic chemicals, called heterocyclic amines (HCAs), are formed from the cooking of muscle meats (including poultry) and they are linked to breast and colon cancer for women and prostate and colon cancer for men. Frying, grilling and barbecuing produce the largest amounts of HCAs because temperature is the most important factor in producing these HCAs. So stewing and poaching have the least effect because of the lower temperature of the cooking method.

In my opinion red meat – beef, pork, lamb and game – should be avoided completely in the fertility-boosting diet.

As for chicken, my biggest concern is regarding quality. The birds' unnatural diets and lack of exercise mean that they actually contain more fat than protein, so should not be seen as a good protein food. Research from the Institute of Brain Chemistry and Human Nutrition at London Metropolitan University has shown that in today's chickens there is 22.8g of fat per 100g compared to 8.6g in 1970 and organic chicken is only slightly better than intensively reared chickens at 17.1g. And that is saturated fat.

My recommendation is that a diet of just fish, eggs, nuts, seeds and legumes would be ideal. If you can't live without meat, poultry is a better choice but limit it to no more than two or three times a week.

PROTEIN SPOT CHECK *Include:* organic fish, eggs, nuts, beans, lentils and seeds. *Avoid:* pies, ready meals, microwave dinners, sausages, hot dogs, burgers, pâtés, red meat, processed meats.

DAIRY PRODUCTS

Dairy products like milk and cheese have traditionally been a mainstay of the Western diet. Some studies[11] indicate that dairy products have a beneficial effect on fertility because of their calcium content, while others[12] have found that in populations where milk consumption is highest, women tend to be less fertile at older ages than non-milk-drinking women. The culprit appears to be lactose, a sugar found in milk that some people can't digest and which could damage human eggs.

My issue with dairy foods is their production and their possible hormonal effect on your body at a time when hormones need to be functioning normally in both partners. A cow only produces milk after giving birth (basically the same as us with breastfeeding), so in order to get a constant supply of milk, two months after giving birth, the cow is artificially inseminated again in order to keep the cycle going. So the cow is being milked while it is pregnant. But pregnancy comes with high levels of hormones, especially oestrogen, and these go into the milk supply and other dairy products. We know that dairy foods increase concentrations of oestrogen in the blood.[13] Organic sheep's and goat's milk products can be less intensively produced which means the hormone content would be lower.

Also the modern trend of buying low-fat dairy foods may not be the best choice. A recent US study[14] found that women who consumed a lot of low-fat dairy products such as skimmed milk were almost twice as likely to suffer period-related fertility problems as those who did not. Dr Jorge Chavarro from the Harvard Medical School in Boston, Massachusetts, who led the study, advised women trying for a baby to substitute high-fat dairy foods for low-fat. Fat is needed to absorb fat-soluble vitamins such as vitamins A, D and E.

It is preferable for you to get your fats from oily fish, eggs, nuts and seeds rather than from full-fat dairy products but the message from this study seems to be that if you are eating dairy products eat them as nature intended, i.e. the whole food.

My general advice would be to reduce the amount of dairy food you are eating anyway. Out of all the dairy foods, the best choice, whether you are tying to get pregnant or not, is yogurt containing the culture lactobacillus acidophilus which can help your body to eliminate hormones it doesn't need any more. If these 'old' hormones aren't eliminated this can create an imbalance which can have a negative effect on your fertility. When yogurts are heated they often lose beneficial bacteria, like lactobacillus acidophilus, so buy yogurts that are 'live' and organic; the label will often read 'bio'. Steer clear of fruit yogurts – they can contain up to eight teaspoons of added sugar. If you avoid dairy foods completely, don't worry about the calcium aspect as your fertility multivitamin and mineral (e.g. Fertility Plus for Women) will contain calcium, as do lots of other foods. You can also take a good probiotic supplement instead of yogurt to get the beneficial bacteria (the one I use in the clinic is BioKult and can be obtained from *www.naturalhealthpractice.com*). If you are concerned you can also be tested to see if you are low in calcium (see mineral test, page 218).

FATS

Unfortunately, fat in general has a bad reputation and many women tend to avoid it as a matter of course, although it is the saturated fats, found in animal meat and the trans fats found in processed food that are harmful and can reduce fertility. Essential fatty acids found in nuts, seeds and oily fish, on the other hand, play a crucial role in fertility and the development of a healthy baby. Scientists have looked at their role in pregnancy and found they are absolutely vital for the developing brain, eyes and nervous system of a growing baby.[15]

If you don't eat enough EFAs, hormone production will also be compromised. It can take up to three months to build up your body's stores, so make sure you eat some every day. Good sources include nuts, seeds, flaxseed (linseed) oil and oily fish. To avoid the consumption of toxins always choose cold-pressed, preferably organic, unrefined nut or seed oil or extra virgin olive oil. You should also eat oily fish such as mackerel or sardines and take an EFA supplement (see Step 3).

Saturated fats are generally harmful because they can cause high cholesterol and increase the risk of heart disease. They also interfere with your body's absorption of EFAs.

Saturated fats which have undergone a chemical process called hydrogenation and are also known as trans fatty acids are the worst culprits and should always be avoided. Found in fried foods, cakes, biscuits, chips and pastries, they interfere with cells involved in ovulation, according to a recent study. The results of research, published in the *American Journal of Clinical Nutrition* showed the chance of becoming pregnant dropped by 73 per cent for every extra 4g of trans fats – the equivalent of half a portion of takeaway fried chicken – eaten each day. Researchers tracked over 18,000 women over eight years and found that those who consumed a high intake of trans fats had an almost 80 per cent chance of having problems with ovulation. Interestingly, consuming polyunsaturated fatty acids (like sunflower, sesame oils) actually reduced the risk of infertility. And because semen is rich in prostaglandins which are made from EFAs it is especially important for men to avoid trans fatty acids too.[16]

You'll often find hydrogenated vegetable oil listed in the ingredients of margarines, shortenings, fried foods, fast foods, processed foods, crisps, biscuits and crackers, so either choose organic butter or unhydrogenated margarine.

UNSATURATED FATS Unsaturated fats are divided into monounsaturated and polyunsaturated fats. Monounsaturated fats, such as olive oil, are thought to lower the risk of heart disease. Polyunsaturated fats (classed as essential fats) can be split into omega 6 oils (found in unrefined sesame, corn and sunflower oils) and omega 3 oils (in fish oils and linseed – or flax – oil). The body makes hormone-regulating substances called prostaglandins from omega 3 and omega 6 oils and they are extremely important for boosting fertility. Symptoms of an essential fatty acid deficiency include: dry skin, dry hair, irritability, brittle nails, fatigue, weight gain, high blood pressure, PMS, arthritis, poor wound healing, hair loss and cracked skin, especially on the heels and fingertips.

FAT SPOT CHECK *Include:* extra virgin olive oil, sunflower oil, sesame oil, nut butters (like almond, cashew), unhydrogenated margarine, butter, fish oils, linseed (flax) oil, mackerel, sardines, nuts, seeds, soya beans, sweet potatoes, walnuts. *Avoid:* red meat, lamb, pork, poultry, hydrogenated margarine, pastries, pies, biscuits, crisps, sweets, ice cream, cereal bars containing hydrogenated fats, deep-fried food.

BENEFITS OF OILY FISH Oily fish are one of the healthiest sources of essential fats – in particular omega 3. And the benefits extend beyond fertility and into pregnancy. A study in the *Lancet* found that women who ate at least 350g of fish a week while pregnant had children who were more advanced in tests measuring motor, communication and social skills and who had better verbal IQ scores. The children of mothers who had eaten little or no fish in pregnancy were 35 per cent more likely to have poor communication skills by the time they were toddlers and the risk of bad behaviour and low verbal IQ at the age of eight was almost 50 per cent higher.[17]

But what about concerns regarding mercury, classed as a heavy toxic metal and which is known, at high levels, to cause brain damage in unborn babies? We're being told on the one hand to eat oily fish for good health and fertility, as well as for the health and intellectual development of your baby. Yet, on the other hand, the Food Standards Agency is telling pregnant women not to eat more than two portions of oily fish a week.

Researchers who looked at the levels of mercury in babies whose mothers ate fish daily checked the umbilical cords and found that even with eating fish once a day, the mercury levels were generally low and confirmed that the babies were more intelligent.[18]

To keep mercury exposure to the minimum, avoid shark, marlin and swordfish when trying to conceive or when pregnant. These fish live a long time so the mercury levels can be more concentrated in them than in other oily fish such as salmon, herring, trout and sardines. Canned fish should be avoided too. Researchers from the Harvard School of Public Health in the US found that women who ate the most canned fish tended to have more mercury in their bodies.[19]

As a general rule, I would suggest eating oily fish once or twice a week but also to take fish oil supplements (not cod liver oil – see page 81) as omega 3 fatty acids are important for healthy brain and eye development in the foetus and also for a healthy birth weight. Make sure that you buy supplements from a reputable company so that you know it has been screened and is free from contaminants (I use a supplement called Omega 3 Plus in the clinic.)

PHYTOESTROGENS

Phytoestrogens are substances found in food which are thought to have a hormone-balancing effect. They may be classified as follows:
~ isoflavones – in legumes such as lentils, soya beans and chick peas
~ lignans – in nearly all grains and vegetables, the best source being flaxseeds
~ coumestans – mainly in alfalfa and mung bean sprouts.

Phytoestrogens are being studied all around the world for their effectiveness in lowering cholesterol and preventing heart disease, but they also play a role in balancing male and female sex hormones.[20]
Note: there has been concern in recent years that eating soya harms female fertility but this is only when consumed in large quantities.[21] Infertility doesn't tend to be a big problem in China or Japan where women regularly eat soya in their daily diet, but they aren't consuming mega doses. So as long as you eat soya no more than five times a week, and choose organic not genetically modified, it will have a positive effect on your fertility.

Research has also suggested that soya could negatively impact on the ability of the sperm to fertilise eggs. However, in my opinion, the way in which this was tested (by exposing sperm to genistein – an isoflavone in soya – in a dish) does not replicate the effects that might be experienced by eating the foods.

Also to take a single isoflavone in isolation, I feel, gives a false picture. And again, with so many cultures around the world eating isoflavones in beans – hummus in the Middle East, dahl (lentils) in Asian countries, soya in Japan – and no signs of a raging fertility problem there really doesn't seem to be cause for alarm.

PRO-FERTILITY NUTRIENTS

The optimum fertility diet recommendations above should ensure an adequate intake of every nutrient, but some nutrients are more essential for your fertility than others. You need only visit your doctor's surgery to see the numerous posters about the importance of folic acid to help prevent neural tube defects like spina bifida, but there are many other vitamins and minerals essential to your reproductive health which can make all the difference to your fertility. The list below suggests the best food sources but for more research and advice about supplementing with specific vitamins and minerals see Step 3, pages 78–90.

Vital vitamins and minerals

Vitamin A: you need good levels of vitamin A at the point of conception because it is essential to the developing embryo and in studies with animals a deficiency of vitamin A produced newborns with birth defects. High doses of vitamin A from animal sources, e.g. liver, are not advised as this can also cause birth defects, but vegetable sources of beta carotene, which your body can turn into vitamin A, are safe.[22] Vitamin A as beta carotene is found in carrots, tomatoes, mangoes, pumpkins, cabbage, egg yolk, parsley, red peppers and broccoli.

Vitamin B6: research has found that eating foods rich in vitamin B6 can more than double your chances of becoming pregnant. It is important for reproductive health, the formation of female sex hormones and regulating oestrogen and progesterone levels. Women who have plenty of vitamin B6 in their diet are also only half as likely to miscarry in the critical first weeks of pregnancy.[23] It is thought that B6 – found in high levels in potatoes, bananas, eggs, peanuts, mushrooms, oats, soya beans, seaweeds, sunflower seeds, salmon and mackerel – plays a key role in the development of the placenta.

Vitamin B12: another B vitamin that is important for your fertility,[24] B12 is found in eggs, seaweeds, sardines and tuna.

Other B vitamins: vitamins B5, B1 and B2 are all essential for a healthy pregnancy. Vitamin B5 or pantothenic acid is found in whole grains, mushrooms, green vegetables, beans, chick peas, soya beans and brown rice; B1 is found in whole grains, beans, peas, lentils, soya beans, eggs and green leafy vegetables; and B2 is in whole grains, green vegetables, eggs, soya beans, peas and mushrooms.

Folic acid: until recently this B vitamin was known mainly for its role in preventing spina bifida in babies but now conclusive research[25] has shown its vital role in fertility.[26] Food sources include green beans, leafy vegetables, broccoli, green peas, asparagus, salmon, alfalfa sprouts, chick peas, oranges, strawberries, bananas, grapefruit and wholemeal bread. However, this is such an important nutrient that all experts recommend taking it as a supplement in the pre-conception period.

Vitamin C: research in the 1970s showed that when given to women undergoing fertility treatment vitamin C could help to trigger ovulation. Recent research is confirming vitamin C's crucial role[27] not just in women but in men. Studies[28] have shown that it can increase sperm count by up to a third. Vitamin C is found in raw fruits and vegetables, especially citrus fruits, blueberries, kiwi fruit, mangoes, red peppers, strawberries, green sprouting vegetables like Brussels sprouts, watercress and parsley.

Vitamin E: this vitamin's beneficial role in female reproductive health has been backed up by recent research.[29] It is required for muscle strength and hormone function and for the metabolism of essential fatty acids and may reduce the risk of miscarriage. It also helps with sperm function.[30] Food sources include cold-pressed unrefined oils, whole grains, egg yolk, green leafy vegetables, avocados, lettuce, peanuts, sesame seeds, soya beans, unrefined cereals, nuts, oily fish, broccoli.

Calcium: this is important for women in general, to keep their bones strong. It helps keep your teeth strong as well, and is necessary for your nervous system and blood clotting. For all of these reasons, it is even more important for a pregnant or trying-to-get-pregnant woman to have adequate calcium so that the baby's teeth, bones, nervous system and blood are all formed properly. Although many of us do rely on milk for our calcium intake always bear in mind that there are many other non-dairy sources, such as sardines, salmon, prunes, almonds, oranges, papayas, watermelon, spinach, nuts, sesame seeds, pulses, leafy green vegetables and whole grains.

Essential fatty acids: see page 81.

Zinc: this mineral is vital for the health and maintenance of reproductive hormones in both men and women.[31] Deficiency in women can lead to reduced fertility and increased risk of miscarriage. It is also vital for the development of unborn babies. Food sources include eggs, apricots, whole grains, dried fruit, seaweed, sunflower seeds, all vegetables, watermelon, mushrooms, beetroot, oily fish, onions, nuts, peas and beans.

Manganese: research has shown[32] that women with low manganese levels are more likely to give birth to a baby with a malformation or to children with behavioural difficulties. Good food sources for manganese include whole grains, seeds, leafy vegetables, sweet potatoes, eggs, onions, green beans, parsley, strawberries, bananas, apples, pineapple, cherries and legumes.

Selenium: selenium deficiency in women has been linked to an increased risk of miscarriage.[33] Good food sources for selenium include herring, tuna, garlic, eggs, carrots, mushrooms, whole wheat, broccoli and garlic.

Magnesium: according to research,[34] magnesium could be one of the most important minerals affecting a woman's ability to conceive and the maintenance of the pregnancy itself. Food sources include dairy products, nuts, green vegetables, eggs, avocado, dried apricots, brown rice, bananas and sunflower seeds.

FOR HIM

Men need to eat a healthy, nutritionally sound diet rich in whole grains, fruits and vegetables, legumes, nuts, seeds and oily fish, including foods rich in vitamins A, B, C and E, zinc, selenium and essential fatty acids.[35]

Modern diets tend to be low in zinc, and stress, pollution, smoking and alcohol all deplete the body's levels further. Zinc is needed for the production of sperm and the male hormones and several prominent research studies have found that the male sex glands and sperm contain high concentrations of zinc.

Vitamin C has been shown to reduce the tendency of sperm to clump together (agglutination), a common factor in infertility.

Researchers from the Shaare Zedek Medical Centre in Jerusalem say that men with infertility consume less omega 3 fatty acids than fertile men. One fatty acid component in particular, alpha linolenic acid, has been shown to have a significant effect on sperm quality and researchers advise men attending fertility clinics to supplement with omega 3 in the belief it will increase low levels of fertility by making the sperm more resistant to potential damage caused by the chilling and freezing processes involved in some assisted-reproduction techniques.

FERTILITY FOODS

Almonds (and nuts in general) and oily fish: prime sources of essential fatty acids; almonds are also a good source of zinc.

Strawberries: a great source of vitamin C; all other fruit and vegetables – particularly kiwi fruit, peppers and citrus fruits – contain abundant quantities of vitamin C.

Green leafy vegetables: good levels of vitamin B6 and folic acid.

Nuts, legumes and whole grains: another great source of folic acid.

Sweet potatoes: a comforting source of manganese.

Sunflower seeds: very good for magnesium.

Water: critical to your fertility. Drinking plenty of water helps to flush out wastes and toxins, keep your body running smoothly and provide proper fluids for conception to occur. Get into the habit of drinking at least six to eight glasses a day.

Avocados, sunflower, safflower oils, nuts and seeds: these all contain high levels of vitamin E.

Oily fish or linseeds (flax): great for essential fats (EFAs).

Lentils: a good unsaturated fat source of healthy protein. Other good sources of protein include quinoa, eggs, vegetables, nuts, seeds and soya products.

VEGETARIANS AND VEGANS

If you don't eat any animal produce make sure you substitute animal protein with beans, nuts and seeds. If you are a vegan (and don't eat any foods derived from animals, including dairy products and eggs) you may be lacking in vitamin B12, which is found primarily in animal products. Vegan sources include seaweeds and yeast extract.

WHAT TO AVOID

Besides avoiding foods such as red meat, non-organic poultry and saturated fats (see pages 18–19, 21), there are others you need to be aware of.

CAFFEINE

Researchers have found that caffeine can have an adverse affect on female fertility, so if you want to conceive it makes sense to cut caffeine out altogether.[36] Drinking more than 300mg a day (two to three cups) may also be associated with miscarriage and increase the risk of stillbirth by around 80 per cent. Additional research[37] suggests that caffeine consumption compounds the negative effects of alcohol consumption on female fertility. Men aren't immune either and studies[38] indicate that problems with sperm health seem greater with increased coffee intake.

Caffeine is found in regular coffee, black tea, green tea, some soft drinks, chocolate and many over-the-counter pharmaceuticals. Tea contains tannin as well as caffeine and tannin blocks the absorption of important minerals so if you drink tea with your meals you are preventing vital nutrients from being absorbed in your digestive tract.

Chocolate contains caffeine too and you can't cheat by switching to organic dark chocolate! It does have less sugar than milk chocolate but its percentage of cocoa solids will be higher, making the caffeine effect even stronger.

Methylxanthines – a family of substances found in coffee, black and green tea, chocolate, cocoa, cola and decaffeinated coffee as well as some medications, such as headache remedies – have been linked to a benign breast condition called fibrocystic disease. Many women experience breast discomfort in the week before a period and for some women this can be very uncomfortable.

While not every study finds that caffeine reduces female fertility, I still recommend cutting back on your intake with a view to eventually avoiding it altogether if you are struggling to get pregnant.

Decaffeinated options for tea and coffee aren't really a good substitute as we have no idea how many chemicals are involved in the decaffeination process. However, you can use them in the weaning stages to get you off the caffeinated drinks. Begin by substituting decaffeinated coffee for half of your total intake a day and then gradually change over to all decaffeinated. Then, slowly substitute again with other drinks, such as herbal teas and grain coffees. You should, ideally, eventually eliminate decaffeinated coffee as well because coffee contains other stimulants (theobromine and theophylline) which are not removed when the coffee is decaffeinated. In one study, drinking three cups of decaffeinated coffee a day was associated with an increased risk of spontaneous abortion.[39]

Experiment with herbal teas. I recommend roasted herbal roots such as barley, chicory and dandelion and lemongrass, peppermint, ginger root, rosehip, apple, hibiscus, clover flower, nettles and chamomile. These can be nourishing and satisfying without the depleting effects of caffeine.

ALCOHOL

This is a complete no-no when it comes to fertility for both men and women. It acts as a diuretic (causing valuable fertility nutrients like zinc and folic acid to be excreted) and a toxin to the sperm and egg and to the baby once you are pregnant (see also page 52).

PROCESSED FOODS

One of the most effective changes you can make is to replace pre-packed foods with fresh, whole foods. My advice is to avoid genetically modified foods, processed, convenience foods with high levels of additives and preservatives; and to protect yourself from pesticides by going organic (see below) and reading food labels. The closer your diet is to nature the better.

Chemicals, pesticides and preservatives used on food are toxins that can interfere with your hormonal health and therefore your fertility, the worst culprits being xenoestrogens – environmental toxins found in pesticides, dairy produce and meat, fish from polluted waters, plastic containers and cling film (see pages 94–105).

ORGANIC

Organic foods often contain higher levels of nutrients and their production is governed by strict standards: pesticides are avoided and animals are raised in natural conditions on organically farmed land and must not be treated with antibiotics. This means that organic food contains less chemical residue than non-organic. If you think it is too expensive, consider buying just one item a week and view it as an investment for your health. You could also get mail order boxes delivered to your door or visit your local farmers' market to get a better deal. Make sure the food you buy is really organic by looking for certification labels from well-respected organisations such as the Soil Association in the UK or Earth Source Greens in the USA.

If, however, going organic isn't practical for you there are still ways in which you can protect yourself against xenoestrogens:

~ Think brown – go for unrefined complex carbohydrates (brown rice, wholemeal pasta, brown bread).
~ Eat a leafy, green vegetable a day. Vegetables such as broccoli, cauliflower or cabbage can boost the liver's ability to detoxify harmful chemicals and hormones.
~ Rinse, don't soak, fresh fruit and vegetables as it's a more effective way to remove pesticide residue. Peel fruit and vegetables before using them. Remove and discard the outer leaves of cabbages and other greens. (If you buy organic you need only scrub the skins.)
~ Eat a wide variety of fruit and vegetables as specific pesticides are used for specific crops – that way you'll avoid too much of a given pesticide.

READING FOOD LABELS

For women who are trying to conceive, additives in the form of colourings, preservatives, flavour enhancers, emulsifiers and thickeners can add to the toxic load and increase the likelihood of hormonal imbalance, irregular periods and weight gain – all of which can have a negative impact on fertility.

Food manufacturers are required to list the ingredients in their products. But how do you decipher a long list of chemical names that look unfamiliar to you? A good general rule is simply to avoid products whose chemical ingredients outnumber the familiar ones or whose labels you can't understand. Also, make sure you check for and avoid artificial sweeteners such as saccharin and aspartame.

With so many chemicals being used today in food products it is not always easy to make the right choices, but if you try to eat food that is as fresh and as natural as possible you are doing fine. If on the odd occasion you need to buy a prepared meal, make sure you choose a good-quality product with a short list of ingredients. Above all, don't get stressed about it; as you'll see in Step 2, stress doesn't help you or your fertility.

HEALTHY SHOPPING CHOICES

The first step towards healthy eating is to select healthy ingredients. Start by throwing out salty convenience foods, fatty food and snacks, sugary drinks and snacks, hydrogenated oils and junk food products from your fridge and cupboards – this can be very liberating! If in doubt about a certain food or drink – get rid of it.

Now it's time to restock your fridge and shelves. Never shop when you are hungry, stressed or tired as your good intentions could crumble in the face of temptation and you'll load your trolley with sugar-rich but nutrient-poor convenience foods. Have a clear idea of what you are going to buy so you are less likely to make unhealthy choices.

Fruit and vegetables Buy organic if you can, specifically peaches, peppers, strawberries, cherries, celery, apples, apricots, green beans, grapes and cucumbers as according to the US FDA (Food and Drug Administration) these foods consistently contain the most pesticides. Dried fruits are a healthy choice but avoid any that contain the preserving agent sulphur dioxide or mineral oil.

Grains If money is limited for buying organic produce, try to buy organic grains because grains tend to absorb more pesticides than other foods as they are smaller.

Bread Organic wholemeal bread, wholemeal pitta bread, rye or spelt bread should be your loaves of choice but do check the labels for undesirable ingredients.

Cereals I recommend sugar-free shredded wheat and puffed rice or wheat or no-added sugar muesli. Soak muesli for ten minutes before eating to break down the phytates, which can block the uptake of minerals from food. Porridge is also a good breakfast cereal (but don't buy the quick-cook or instant variety because its speed of cooking means that it is absorbed into the bloodstream faster and is therefore not a slow-releasing carbohydrate).

Flavourings Avoid processed flavourings and instead choose from fresh and dried herbs, ginger, lemon juice, miso (soya bean paste), mustard and arrowroot for thickening to make sauces or gravies. Soya sauce is good for salads and stir-fries but avoid any that contains monosodium glutamate. Tamari, wheat-free soya sauce, is also good. Some ready-made salad dressings with no chemicals or sugar are worth a try too.

Salt Get out of the habit of buying salt. Use herbs and spices, lemon juice, vinegar, onions, garlic and chillies instead. A diet high in salt can increase your risk of high blood pressure and fluid retention. If you're addicted to salt try a salt substitute such as LoSalt which contains potassium instead of sodium. You also need to be aware that salt is a hidden ingredient in many foods so read labels to check for the salt (sodium) content. You should be aiming for no more than 5g of salt a day.

Sweeteners It is always best to use natural sweeteners, such as fruit or raisins, rather than sugar or artificial sweeteners. Honey is fine in moderation but make sure you avoid those that are blended or heated to high temperatures as they are processed and therefore higher in sugar and additives than pure honey from one source. Maple syrup is also an option but make sure it is the real maple syrup and not 'maple-flavoured syrup'.

Beans/pulses These are an important part of your fertility-boosting diet because they will often be used to replace meat. Hummus, which is made from chick peas, can be bought ready made from supermarkets. Most beans need to be soaked overnight before cooking or you could buy organic tinned varieties, like kidney beans.

Meat If you are eating meat, poultry (such as chicken and turkey) would be the better choice and, if you can, try to get organic, free-range or corn-fed birds. It's best to avoid red meat completely (see page 18) but if you do eat it the government recommends no more than 95g a day.

Fish Choose oily fish such as mackerel, tuna, salmon, sardines and anchovies. Fresh and frozen are best. Grill or poach fish rather than frying it.

Dairy produce If you can, go for dairy produce that is organic and free of antibiotics and chemicals. If you are intolerant to milk try goat's or sheep's milk or drink organic soya, rice or oat milk which can also be used in cooking. Buy live yogurt containing the culture lactobacillus acidophilus – organic if possible. That way you reduce your intake of chemicals that can inhibit your fertility (see pages 19–20).

Soya Buy organic soya that is not genetically modified and if you buy soya milk make sure it is sugar-free. Soya bean curd, also known as tofu, can be used in stir-fries, soups and desserts; again buy organic and GM-free. Avoid any products made from soya protein isolate as the process used to make it leaves traces of aluminium and nitrates. Up to 60 per cent of processed foods contain soya (including bread, biscuits, pizza and baby food) and in the majority of cases the soya takes the form of soya isolate, and is not derived from whole soya beans, so be aware of this when checking labels.

Oils Use butter (organic if possible) and unhydrogenated margarines. Look for cold-pressed, unrefined vegetable oils like sunflower and sesame and use extra virgin olive oil for light cooking.

Drinks Try grain coffees, like Caro and Bambu, which contain various combinations of ingredients like barley and rye, and experiment with herbal teas, fruit teas and Rooibos. Check the labels on fruit juices and avoid any that say 'fruit drink' or 'fruit juice drink' as that means they contain sugar and additives. Watch out for flavoured waters as they can contain sugar. If you want to buy bottled water for drinking bear in mind that spring water has undergone filtration and blending, natural mineral water is bottled in its natural mineral state without treatment, natural sparkling water is natural water from its underground source with enough carbon dioxide naturally occurring to make it bubbly and carbonated water has carbon dioxide added during bottling. Choose glass rather than plastic bottles to reduce exposure to xenoestrogens (see page 95).

SUMMARY

For the optimum fertility-boosting diet cut out caffeine, reduce your intake of saturated fats, white flour products, sugar, processed foods, red meat and unhealthy snacks, crisps and sweets. Instead, eat a diet rich in organic vegetables, fruit, fish, nuts, seeds, beans, pulses and whole-grain products. Drink six to eight glasses of water a day (try starting each day with a cup of warm water and a slice of lemon – it's so refreshing and is excellent for digestion). Going organic and choosing foods based on the information on their labels will also dramatically increase your chances of conception.

Here's an 'at-a-glance checklist' to stick on your fridge:

Whole grains: eat every day, including brown rice, whole wheat and oats.

Fruit and vegetables: three to five servings of vegetables a day and two to three servings of fruit a day. (One serving of fruit is one medium whole fruit, 115g cooked or tinned fruit (in juice not syrup) or 100g fruit juice. One serving of vegetables is 145g raw, leafy vegetables and 115g of other vegetables.)

Protein: aim for around two to three servings of fish, beans, eggs or nuts a day. (One serving is 60–90g cooked fish, 115g beans, 1 egg or 100g nuts.)

Dairy: look for organic dairy products and limit your intake. (One serving is 240ml milk or yogurt or 45g cheese.)

Fats: avoid hydrogenated vegetable oils and use cold-pressed, unrefined vegetable oils – around 5–7 teaspoons a day, made up of different oils, such as sunflower, sesame and extra virgin olive oil.

Water: drink at least six to eight glasses a day.

OTHER NUTRITION-RELATED FACTORS

Now that the basics of healthy eating for fertility have been explained let's look at other nutrition-related factors that you need to be aware of.

CONTROLLING BLOOD SUGAR LEVELS

The amount of sugar (glucose) that is circulating in your bloodstream can have a huge impact on your fertility. Blood sugar levels start to climb every time you eat and your body then produces insulin in response to move the sugar into your cells to be used for energy. If you eat the kind of foods recommended in my pre-conception diet – whole grains, vegetables and fruit, nuts, seeds, oily fish and legumes – these are digested and absorbed slowly and your blood sugar levels and insulin levels will rise and fall gradually within the normal range. If, however, you eat too many sugary and processed foods, e.g. white bread and cakes, your blood sugar and insulin levels can shoot up faster and faster – well above the normal range. If this continues too much insulin is produced and this will unsettle your reproductive hormones and hinder ovulation.

Overproduction of insulin – and a resulting condition called insulin resistance – lies at the root of many problems which hinder fertility, including obesity, polycystic ovarian syndrome (PCOS) and diabetes, but even if you don't have insulin resistance a diet based on whole foods or foods that are low on the glycaemic index (GI) – meaning that they are absorbed and digested slowly – is a good idea for both your health and your fertility. This is because swings in blood sugar can spark off sugar cravings and bingeing habits that make you eat the wrong foods and put on weight.

In addition, if your blood sugar levels frequently drop your body will start to pump out more of the stress hormone adrenaline. When this happens your liver immediately releases emergency stores of glucose into your system and your digestion shuts down to give you instant energy to fight or run in response to stress. The trouble is there is often no outside stress to respond to and these surges of adrenaline can contribute to heart disease by increasing the risk of high blood pressure. And as far as your fertility is concerned the release of adrenaline can also block your body's ability to utilise the reproductive hormone progesterone, essential for maintaining pregnancy.

So controlling blood sugar levels is crucial for hormone balance and for your fertility and the best way to do that is to adjust your diet accordingly.

Your blood sugar levels rise and fall depending on two main factors: what you eat and when you eat or drink.

When you eat refined food you digest it very fast because refined foods have been stripped of their natural goodness by the manufacturing process. Two of the most common refined foods are white flour and sugar. When digestion is too fast you get a sharp rise in blood sugar giving you a temporary lift. But the initial high will soon plummet leaving you tired and drained when your blood sugar levels drop again. When this happens you may experience cravings for a bar of chocolate or a coffee and a vicious cycle is set up that can cause an up and down rollercoaster of blood sugar swings and hormonal chaos.

Whole foods, however, such as complex carbohydrates, are absorbed slowly into your bloodstream so that you avoid blood sugar swings and the negative effects they have on your mood, health and fertility.

If you leave more than three hours between meals and snacks your blood glucose will drop to a low level making you more likely to crave sweet foods that can give you a quick boost. If, however, you eat little and often and develop a grazing mentality you keep your blood sugar levels constant and food cravings at bay. That's why my pre-conception diet advises that you try not to leave more than three hours without eating. Many of us find ourselves skipping breakfast or grabbing a coffee, followed by a light lunch and then an evening meal, maybe as late as 9 or 10pm. Starving and stacking your calories like this isn't a good idea if you are trying for a baby. Not to mention the fact that if you leave long periods between meals your body thinks starvation is on the menu and responds by doing its best to hold onto every calorie by reducing your metabolism and preparing to store fat.

So, to balance your blood sugar levels you need to eat more often and eat complex carbohydrates rather than refined foods, especially sugar.

HEALTHY SNACKING IDEAS

~ Crisp, raw vegetables cut up (celery, carrots, cauliflower, broccoli, green pepper, green beans, cucumber, mushrooms, courgettes) and served with a healthy dip like hummus.

~ Celery sticks, 6–8 cm long, filled with cottage cheese and topped with sultanas or chopped nuts.

~ Handful of nuts and/or seeds with fresh fruit in season, cut in slices or halves (apples, oranges, bananas, peaches, grapefruit, grapes, melons, pears, plums or strawberries).

~ A mixture of nuts and dried fruits.

~ Whole wheat, rye, spelt or oat crackers spread with mashed banana and cinnamon, or try mashed avocado, sliced tomato and sprouting seeds.

~ Chopped hard-boiled egg served with sugar-free mayonnaise, herbs and spices on a cracker.

~ Plain live organic yogurt topped with nuts and seeds.

~ A round of pitta bread with tomato paste and herbs, topped with tomato and hummus (add onion, sliced mushrooms or pineapple).

~ A little organic Cheddar cheese sprinkled over wholemeal pitta bread. Grill to make a tasty pizza.

~ Fruity kebabs: bite-size pieces of fruit in season on kebab skewers and sprinkled with seeds.

HOW TO CUT BACK ON YOUR SUGAR INTAKE

~ Take the sugar bowl off the table.

~ Avoid sweets, biscuits, cakes, pies, doughnuts and other processed, refined foods with added sugar.

~ Look out for sugar in pre-packaged foods from cheese slices to breakfast cereals, tomato sauces, baked beans and soups.

~ Eat fresh fruit or toasted rye bread with pure fruit jam (sugar-free, not diabetic or with artificial sweeteners).

~ Go for oat or whole-grain breakfast cereals that have no added sugar.

~ Beware of any word in an ingredient list ending in '-ose' e.g. fructose (fruit sugar), glucose (fast acting), dextrose (from cornstarch, chemically identical to glucose), lactose (milk sugar), maltose (from starch), sucrose (common table sugar, made from sugar cane or beet).

SUGAR – BY ANY OTHER NAME Food companies are obliged to put the main ingredient (i.e. the one in greatest quantity) first on the list. If all sugars were grouped under the word 'sugar' this word would appear first in countless foods. However, they split sugar into its different forms to spread the perceived sugar load and shift it a little further down the list. So start reading the labels on your favourite foods more carefully and you will find it in one of its many guises: sucrose, raw sugar, brown sugar, muscovado sugar, turbinado sugar, sucrose, dextrose, honey, lactose, invert sugar, confectioner's sugar, corn syrup, fructose, glucose, sorbitol, mannitol, malitol, treacle, molasses. The list goes on.

But is any of these sugars better than the others? The bottom line is 'sugar is sugar' and in any form it's high in calories and low in nutrients. Sugar substitutes and sweeteners aren't much better either as they've been linked to stomach upsets, hormonal problems, headaches and even weight gain and cancer.

FOOD ALLERGIES

Fertility can suffer if you have a food allergy (to milk, wheat, etc.). Such allergies (also known as intolerances) can thicken your cervical mucus, making it harder for sperm to reach the egg. In men they may also thicken sperm and diminish its ability to fertilise.

Treating a food allergy is outside the scope of this book, but if you have any of these symptoms it is possible that you are suffering from a reaction to something you are eating:

~ bloating

~ excess wind (flatulence)

~ diarrhoea

~ constipation

~ heartburn

~ chronic infections

~ skin problems like itching, rashes, eczema, etc.

~ fatigue

~ joint and muscle pains

~ arthritis

~ headaches/migraines

~ rhinitis (constant runny nose)

~ sinus problems.

Keep a food diary and record everything you eat and how you feel after. For example, if you feel bloated and lethargic after eating bread you may have a wheat allergy and if you feel congested after drinking milk you may have a dairy allergy. Try eliminating any suspects for a while and see what happens but do bear in mind that it may take up to three days for allergy symptoms to hit after you have eaten the food. If your diary isn't giving you any clues it might be wise to have a food allergy blood test that measures your reactions to 233 different foods, seasonings, colourings, additives and drinks from one single blood sample. (See page 218 or *www.naturalhealthpractice.com*.)

POOR DIGESTION

Your gut is colonised by bacteria – both good and bad – which must be in balance for good digestive health. Unfortunately, if your diet is poor and stress levels are high this balance is likely to be upset and a poorly recognised but extremely common condition, called leaky gut syndrome, may develop. A leaky gut is bad news for your fertility for a number of reasons. Not only can it cause stomach upsets, bloating, constipation and diarrhoea, it can also trigger a lethal combination of nutritional deficiencies and toxic overload, increasing the likelihood of blood sugar swings and weight gain which, in turn, can trigger hormonal imbalances and fertility problems.

When the gut becomes leaky a compromised intestinal barrier prevents the gut from functioning as a digestive/absorptive organ as well as a barrier to toxic compounds and partially digested food particles. It is thought that increased gut permeability may trigger the start of autoimmune problems, where the body starts to attack its own tissue. This is particularly important in the area of fertility because of the effect of the immune system on getting and staying pregnant. When you think that half of the DNA in a pregnancy is not your own but your partner's, your immune system has to 'dampen' down so that it doesn't reject your pregnancy as it would any other foreign substance like a bacteria. So an overactive immune system is certainly not an advantage when trying to get pregnant (see page 167).

Digestion consists of three processes – absorption, assimilation and excretion; following my pre-conception diet guidelines and making sure you eat enough fibre and drink enough water will keep all this in good working order.

DIGESTION-BOOSTING TIPS

~ *Chew it over:* if you don't chew your food properly you give more work to the rest of the system which puts it under stress. As well as making food easier to swallow, saliva contains enzymes that contribute to the chemical process of digestion. If food is not properly chewed nutrients remain locked in and undigested matter feeds bad bacteria, which can lead to bacterial overgrowth, wind and other symptoms of indigestion. Chewing also relaxes the lower stomach muscle and triggers nerve messages to activate the whole digestive process. Aim to chew food until it is small enough to swallow easily. Remember, how you eat is as important as what you eat for a healthy digestion.

~ *Keep your portions moderate* so your stomach doesn't get stretched and overworked.

~ *Try to eat at regular times:* your digestion system works best when it knows what to expect.

~ *Good bacteria:* probiotics are the good guys, the healthy gut bacteria which are important for the assimilation of nutrients. They create the right environment in your digestive system. A number of factors can disrupt the balance of bacteria in your gut, such as stress, illness (especially diarrhoea), thrush and antibiotics. If you have a hectic lifestyle, are prone to colds, are taking antibiotics or have a history of stress-related digestive disorders such as IBS you could benefit from probiotics. Cultured or fermented foods such as live yogurt also contain various types and amounts. Avoid the well-advertised 'friendly bacteria' drinks, they are often loaded with sugar which just adds to the problem you're trying to solve.

~ *Keep active:* regular aerobic activity (at least 30 minutes of any activity that makes you feel slightly breathless and sweaty five or six days a week) stimulates the muscles of the digestive system, helping you to digest food better and expel waste more efficiently. (See also Step 2, pages 44–77.)

~ *Calm down:* it is important to eat in a relaxed and calm state. Your stomach and intestines are very sensitive to stress and when you feel anxious digestion shuts down to let your body focus on preparing the flight-and-fight response. This leads to poor digestion and eventually certain vitamin and mineral deficiencies. Finding ways to manage and cope with stress is important for your digestive as well as your emotional and reproductive health. (See also Step 2, pages 44–77.)

PCOS, ENDOMETRIOSIS AND FIBROIDS

It has been proved that a change in diet can significantly reduce the symptoms of PCOS, endometriosis and fibroids and increase fertility. It is thought that these conditions are all caused by imbalances in hormones and switching to a low-carbohydrate, high-fibre way of eating can help maintain a healthy blood sugar level and keep hormones in balance. The diet recommendations if you have these conditions follow much the same principles as my pre-conception diet but there are additional requirements you do need to bear in mind. For self-help advice and details of foods to avoid and supplements to take if you have any of these conditions refer to Step 7.

YOUR WEIGHT

Did you know that weight also plays a significant role in fertility? If you are overweight or underweight, your body may be having trouble regulating its natural cycle. You need to be the right weight in order to produce the appropriate amount of hormones to regulate ovulation and menstruation. If not, your body can start to experience problems with these natural fertility cycles, impacting on your ability to become pregnant. In fact, more than 12 per cent of all infertility patients suffer from weight-related infertility.

Research[40] shows that women who are underweight are at risk of compromising their fertility cycle.

Evidence[41] has also recently emerged about reduced fertility in overweight women. It appears the risk of infertility increases with the degree of obesity: in other words, the greater the weight, the bigger the problem. One study[42] showed that when overweight, infertile women successfully followed a weight-loss and exercise programme for six months, their periods returned and most went on to have healthy babies. This is because women who are overweight tend to have a higher percentage of fat on their bodies and as fat cells produce oestrogen, some overweight women produce levels of oestrogen that are far too high. This can negatively influence menstruation and ovulation, making it difficult to become pregnant. Studies[43] have also shown that being significantly overweight may also affect responses to certain fertility treatments, such as IVF. Gaining too much weight between pregnancies can also have a negative impact on fertility and the strong link between infertility and obesity is currently the focus of a great deal of research.[44]

It is not only being the right body weight that is critical for fertility, the amount of body fat you have is just as important. In normal adult women, fat comprises about 28 per cent of body weight and if it drops below 22 per cent ovulation could stop. Women with an average or above average body weight, or who exercise very rigorously, may have a lower body fat and a higher muscle content, which may lead to their periods becoming irregular or stopping altogether. Sensible advice for these women would be to reduce their exercise until their body fat returns to the normal range. Many gyms have simple devices that can check your body fat level or you can buy a fat percentage machine for the price of a good set of bathroom scales.

The most commonly accepted measure of whether or not someone is over or underweight is the Body Mass Index (BMI). Your BMI is the ratio of your height to your weight and is calculated as follows: BMI = your weight in kg divided by the square of your height in metres. For instance if your weight is 63.5kg and your height 1.68m, your BMI would be: $63.5 \div 1.68^2 = 22.5$. So you have a BMI of 22.

If your BMI is under 20 you are considered underweight; if it is between 20 and 25 you are considered normal; between 25 and 30 is overweight; between 30 and 40 is obese and over 40 dangerously obese.

The BMI is a useful tool, but it can't tell the difference between fat and muscle. Because of the way it is calculated a healthy athletic person (with low body fat and lots of muscle) can have the same BMI as a couch potato (whose weight is mostly made up of fat), so it's worth getting a reading for your fat percentage too (see above).

If you're underweight
If your BMI is under 20 you may have problems conceiving and the risk of miscarriage is higher than normal. The theory is that your body does not have enough fat stores to sustain a pregnancy and so ovulation is shut down. When you gain enough weight your body senses that fat stores are more plentiful and pregnancy is a viable option and you become fertile again.

This is one of the major reasons why dieting is not recommended if you are trying for a baby. Research[45] shows that even when healthy women were put on a diet of 1,000 calories a day their periods became irregular because progesterone and oestrogen levels dropped significantly. Another study[46] showed that only 27 per cent of women on a low-fat diet were actually ovulating. Fortunately, gaining weight can restore fertility back to normal and other studies[47] show that nearly three quarters of women with unexplained infertility managed to get pregnant once they stopped dieting and returned to a healthy weight.

Aim for a BMI of between 20 and 25 (the optimum being 24). When you get your weight back to normal (through a diet that includes plenty of whole grains, vegetables, fruit, oily fish, nuts and seeds) I strongly advise you to wait three to four months before trying for a baby as it is highly likely that you may have nutritional deficiencies as a result of previous restricted food intake.

USE THS CHART TO FIND YOUR BODY MASS INDEX

Height in centimetres

Weight in kilograms / **Weight in stones and pounds**

	142	145	147	150	152	155	158	160	163	165	168	170	173	175	178	180	183	
40	20	19	19	18	17	17	16	16	15	15	14	14	13	13	13	12	12	6st 4
41	20	20	19	18	18	17	16	16	15	15	15	14	14	13	13	13	12	6st 6
42	21	20	19	19	18	17	17	16	16	15	15	15	14	14	13	13	13	6st 9
43	21	20	20	19	19	18	17	17	17	16	16	15	15	14	14	13	13	6st 11
44	22	21	20	20	19	18	18	17	17	16	16	15	15	14	14	14	13	6st 13
45	22	21	21	20	19	19	18	18	17	17	16	16	15	15	14	14	13	7st 1
46	23	22	21	20	20	19	18	18	17	17	16	16	15	15	15	14	14	7st 3
47	23	22	22	21	20	20	19	18	18	17	17	16	16	15	15	15	14	7st 6
48	24	23	22	21	21	20	19	19	18	18	17	17	16	16	15	15	14	7st 8
49	24	23	23	22	21	20	20	19	18	18	17	17	16	16	15	15	15	7st 10
50	25	24	23	22	22	21	20	20	19	18	18	17	17	16	16	15	15	7st 12
51	25	24	24	23	22	21	20	20	19	19	18	18	17	17	16	16	15	8st
52	26	25	24	23	23	22	21	20	20	19	18	18	17	17	16	16	16	8st 3
53	26	25	25	24	23	22	21	21	20	19	19	18	18	17	17	16	16	8st 5
54	27	26	25	24	23	22	22	21	20	20	19	19	18	18	17	17	16	8st 7
55	27	26	25	24	24	23	22	21	21	20	19	19	18	18	17	17	16	8st 9
56	28	27	26	25	24	23	22	22	21	21	20	19	19	18	18	17	17	8st 11
57	28	27	26	25	25	24	23	22	21	21	20	20	19	19	18	18	17	9st
58	29	28	27	26	25	24	23	23	22	21	21	20	19	19	18	18	17	9st 2
59	29	28	27	26	26	25	24	23	22	22	21	20	20	19	19	18	18	9st 4
60	30	29	28	27	26	25	24	23	23	22	21	21	20	20	19	19	18	9st 6
61	30	29	28	27	26	25	24	24	23	22	22	21	20	20	19	19	18	9st 9
62	31	29	29	28	27	26	25	24	23	23	22	21	21	20	20	19	19	9st 11
63	31	30	29	28	27	26	25	25	24	23	22	22	21	21	20	19	19	9st 13
64	32	30	30	28	28	27	26	25	24	24	23	22	21	21	20	20	19	10st 1
65	32	31	30	29	28	27	26	25	24	24	23	22	22	21	21	20	19	10st 3
66	33	31	31	29	29	27	26	26	25	24	23	23	22	22	21	20	20	10st 6
67	33	32	31	30	29	28	27	26	25	25	24	23	22	22	21	21	20	10st 8
68	34	32	31	30	29	28	27	27	26	25	24	24	23	22	21	21	20	10st 10
69	34	33	32	31	30	29	28	27	26	25	24	24	23	23	22	21	21	10st 12
70	35	33	32	31	30	29	28	27	26	26	25	24	23	23	22	22	21	11st
71	35	34	33	32	31	30	28	28	27	26	25	25	24	23	22	22	21	11st 3
72	36	34	33	32	31	30	29	28	27	26	26	25	24	24	23	22	21	11st 5
73	36	35	34	32	32	30	29	29	27	27	26	25	24	24	23	23	22	11st 7
74	37	35	34	33	32	31	30	29	28	27	26	26	25	24	23	23	22	11st 9
75	37	36	35	33	32	31	30	29	28	28	27	26	25	24	24	23	22	11st 11
76	38	36	35	34	33	32	30	30	29	28	27	26	25	25	24	23	23	12st
77	38	37	36	34	33	32	31	30	29	28	27	27	26	25	24	24	23	12st 2
78	39	37	36	35	34	32	31	30	29	29	28	27	26	26	25	24	23	12st 4
79	39	38	37	35	34	33	32	31	30	29	28	27	26	26	25	24	24	12st 6
80	40	38	37	36	35	33	32	31	30	29	28	28	27	26	25	25	24	12st 8
81	40	39	37	36	35	34	32	32	30	30	29	28	27	26	26	25	24	12st 11
82	41	39	38	36	35	34	33	32	31	30	29	28	27	27	26	25	24	12st 13
83	41	39	38	37	36	35	33	32	31	30	29	29	28	27	26	26	25	13st 1
84	42	40	39	37	36	35	34	33	32	31	30	29	28	27	27	26	25	13st 3
85	42	40	39	38	37	35	34	33	32	31	30	29	28	28	27	26	25	13st 5
86	43	41	40	38	37	36	34	34	32	32	30	30	29	28	27	27	26	13st 8
87	43	41	40	39	38	36	35	34	33	32	31	30	29	28	27	27	26	13st 10
88	44	42	41	39	38	37	35	34	33	32	31	30	29	29	28	27	26	13st 12
89	44	42	41	40	39	37	36	35	33	33	32	31	30	29	28	27	27	14st
90	45	43	42	40	39	37	36	35	34	33	32	31	30	29	28	28	27	14st 2
	4ft 8	4ft 9	4ft 10	4ft 11	5ft 0	5ft 1	5ft 2	5ft 3	5ft 4	5ft 5	5ft 6	5ft 7	5ft 8	5ft 9	5ft 10	5ft 11	6ft	

Height in feet and inches

Imperial measures given are only approximates

If you are overweight

A BMI of over 25 could have a negative impact on fertility. Studies[48] have shown, however, that just losing a small amount of weight, say 10 per cent, can be enough to trigger ovulation, make your periods more regular and increase fertility.

More often than not changing your diet to one that is nutritious and healthy as recommended in my fertility-boosting diet plan is enough to kick-start weight loss. The advice on pages 33–35 for controlling your blood sugar will also help as there is a clear link between excess weight and the way your blood sugar levels affect your metabolism and ability to lose weight.

To sum up, if you are trying to lose weight all the advice in this chapter is relevant to you. But remember not to get carried away with losing weight as dieting or drastic weight loss have a negative effect on fertility. Try for a gradual weight loss of no more than 900g (1lb) a week – it may not sound much but it soon adds up – and aim to get into your ideal weight range, not at the bottom of it. Snack on healthy foods throughout the day to keep your blood sugar levels on an even keel and food cravings at bay and don't eat big meals after 8pm.

A good night's sleep is important too as lack of sleep disrupts hormones, triggering changes in metabolism so that you're not processing food as well as you could. *Note:* an increasing number of studies[49] show that cinnamon contains substances which can help the body to convert sugar into energy so it's less likely to be stored as fat. Sprinkle it on porridge, where you would normally have added sugar if you want something to make it more interesting.

Remember there may also be other factors at work affecting your weight. Weight gain can be due to water retention – if this is the case drink more water and cut down on salt. Also, if you feel that stress and/or emotional eating is your underlying issue refer to Step 2 (pages 44–77).

THE 80/20 RULE The aim is to eat well 80 per cent of the time so that the occasional blip (the other 20 per cent), such as a birthday party or holiday, doesn't matter. It is what you do every day that counts.

Your partner's weight

Being overweight can affect male fertility too, reducing the quality and quantity of his sperm count. Both overweight and obese men have reduced fertility and obese men have decreased sperm quality.[50] Obviously when both the man and woman are overweight this can have a combined effect on fertility but interestingly in one Danish study there were problems even if only the male partner was overweight.[50]

MY TOP TEN GOLDEN FERTILITY-BOOSTING DIET RULES

This chapter will have helped you to see food as a powerful tool. Not only can it give you energy, lift your mood and help you think more clearly, it can boost your health and your fertility. A delicious and healthy, varied diet is one of life's great pleasures and you deserve to enjoy every tasty mouthful of it. So, remember:

1 Drink plenty of water.
2 Go for high-fibre whole foods (see page 16).
3 Eat plenty of vegetables and fruit.
4 Eat good-quality protein with every meal (see page 18).
5 Eat good amounts of essential oils (see page 21).
6 Always eat breakfast and stop eating after 8pm.
7 Keep your blood sugar levels balanced by eating little and often – every three hours.
8 Eliminate caffeine and sugar.
9 Choose organic food where possible.
10 Reduce or, ideally, eliminate your intake of red meat, saturated fat, convenience foods, refined foods and foods high in additives and preservatives.

step two
changing your lifestyle

Do you wake up in the morning with a spring in your step or do you crawl reluctantly out of bed feeling exhausted and run down before the day even begins? Do you hardly ever get ill or do you always go down with colds or infections? Can you walk or jog without getting out of breath or do you suffer from aches and pains that slow you down? If it's the latter in each instance, these can all be signals that your health, and therefore your fertility, is not at optimum level.

The pre-conception period is the ideal time for you and your partner to focus on your general health and well-being. Eating healthily may be all that you need to do to get back on track but if you don't feel as fit and as well as you possibly can it's time to take a long, good look at lifestyle factors that may be negatively influencing your health and fertility.

Note: this chapter will help you to review these factors but if you know that your health isn't what it should be it is also important to visit your doctor for a general check-up (see pages 110–118 in Step 5 for information on what this check-up should include).

EVERYTHING TO GAIN

One argument I've heard many times against changing diet and lifestyle in order to get pregnant faster is that there are so many people out there who smoke and drink to excess and yet still manage to get pregnant. Quite simply, everyone is different.

If you are not getting pregnant – and especially if you have been given a diagnosis of unexplained infertility – it's clear that something is preventing pregnancy. By making small changes in your lifestyle you can make a huge difference to your fertility. And the fact is, we know it works.

According to one study, couples with more than four negative lifestyle variables (including smoking, alcohol, tea/coffee) took seven times longer to get pregnant.[1] With the number of babies born with defects that may be linked to the mother's diet and lifestyle choices before and during pregnancy having risen by up to 50 per cent in four years, the Birth Defects Foundation is warning women to make lifestyle changes *before* they get pregnant. One in 16 babies in Britain is now born with a defect ranging from spina bifida to cleft lips.

The evidence in favour of a link between lifestyle and fertility is so overwhelming that a study recently published in the medical journal *Human Reproduction Update* states categorically: 'It is concluded that lifestyle modification CAN assist couples to conceive spontaneously or optimise their chances of conception with assisted reproductive technology.'[2]

So by changing your diet and lifestyle over three months you will not only be giving yourself the chance to get pregnant but also to stay pregnant, have a healthy pregnancy and a healthy baby. There is nothing to lose and everything to gain.

THE AGE ISSUE – HOW LONG WILL YOU BE FERTILE?

More and more women are having babies later in life. UK figures for 2003 show that 49 per cent of births were to women aged 30 plus, compared to 20 years ago when this was just 27 per cent. The average age of all mothers giving birth is now 31, the highest ever. But even though 40 is becoming the new 30 (or 20 even) and women are living longer and feeling and looking younger, the undeniable truth is that the biological clock still ticks away at the same rate it did a generation ago and a woman is still considered to be in her reproductive prime in her 20s. Past the age of 35 the clock speeds up, making it more difficult to conceive, even if you are trying for your second or third child.

At around the age of 35 most women start to become less fertile and may not ovulate every month, even though their periods are still regular. (A slight shortening of the monthly menstrual cycle is also common with age.) So if you have problems conceiving, being over 35 isn't going to boost your chances, but try not to let this panic you. Whatever your age you can still raise your fertility levels with diet and lifestyle changes and, if needed, fertility treatment.

The trouble is that women who delay motherhood can be unwittingly pushing themselves towards infertility and thinking that IVF is a fallback. This unfortunately, however, has a high failure rate (75 per cent of cycles fail in the UK and USA, rising to 90 per cent over the age of 40). The other problem is that everybody's biological clock is different and for some women their clock, or egg reserve, runs down much faster than the average woman without them even knowing.

YOUR EGG RESERVE

Your store of eggs is already in place when you are born. Most women are born with about 2 million egg follicles; by puberty there are about 750,000 and by the age of around 45 there may only be 10,000 left. Of course, that means that at the age of 35 those eggs are older than they were when you were 25.

Each month during your menstrual cycle, about 20 eggs are developing ready for ovulation but only one or two win the race. These are the 'good' eggs. As you get older the chances of having 'good' eggs gets less because the eggs are older and more prone to chromosomal defects which can either prevent fertilisation in the first place or increase the risk of a miscarriage.

TESTING FOR OVARIAN RESERVE

As you are born with a set supply of eggs, a test that can show you how many eggs you have in store and, more importantly, how much time you have left can be helpful because the difference between chronological age and biological clock age can vary enormously. One way to do this is to go for ultrasound testing during the first half of the cycle. This test examines the size of a woman's ovaries and the number of measurable small (antral) follicles (developing eggs). Another test which is more convenient (because it does not require an appointment with a clinic and also does not depend on the time of the month) is a blood test to measure a hormone called Anti-mullerian hormone (AMH). Called a 'new marker for ovarian function',[3] AMH is made by the ovaries and helps the eggs mature each month. It is also important in the production of the female sex hormone oestrogen. The level of AMH indicates how well your ovaries are functioning and represents both the quantity and quality of the egg store.[4] The lower the level of AMH the lower the fertility level is likely to be. This is a useful test also if you are thinking about doing IVF as it has been used in clinical trials to predict poor response to IVF treatment.[5] In order for IVF or ICSI to work, your ovaries have to respond to the drug stimulation by recruiting a group of follicles, so if AMH is low then it is more than likely that the response will be poor.

Measuring AMH is also useful for women with suspected polycystic ovary syndrome (PCOS) as the level is normally very high due to the greater number of follicles on the ovaries.

Another fertility test is to measure levels of FSH (follicle-stimulating hormone). FSH is released from the pituitary gland and its role is to stimulate a group of follicles to grow on the surface of the ovary. So FSH should be low at the beginning of the cycle because it is only just beginning to rise. If the FSH level is high at this time, it means that the ovaries need more stimulation in order to grow follicles for ovulation. This can be a reflection of ovarian reserve because if there are fewer eggs, the pituitary gland has got to release more FSH in order to stimulate those eggs; in effect the body has to work harder to ovulate.

In January 2006 a new home test, called the Plan Ahead test, was launched in the UK to help women find out for themselves how many eggs are left in their ovaries. The Plan Ahead test (see page 218) works by measuring the levels of hormones in blood, taken in the early part of a woman's cycle. The woman's estimated ovarian reserve is given compared to an average woman of that age. The test was developed by Professor Bill Ledger from the University of Sheffield, who hopes that the test 'will help many women avoid the anguish caused by the early or unexpected arrival of declining fertility and menopause'.

The problem with all of these tests is that they measure the quantity not the quality of the eggs, and when you are trying to get pregnant the quality does matter. The consensus, therefore, is that AMH is a better marker for ovarian reserve than FSH and is even more consistent as a marker than ultrasound antral follicle count.[6]

It is not possible to change the quantity of eggs you have and if you have found out that your egg reserve is low then you may need to think about the other options available such as egg donation, surrogacy or adoption. But if you are still having periods and ovulating most months, it is possible that by following my fertility-boosting diet and lifestyle recommendations you can change the *quality* of your eggs to give you the best chance of conceiving naturally and preventing a miscarriage.

YOUR PARTNER'S AGE

For many years it was thought that age only mattered with women when it came to fertility but we now know that the man's age counts too.

Men do have a biological clock and, like women's, it starts ticking around the age of 35. Research has shown that with men over the age of 35 the count is lower and the sperm are less motile and the risk of miscarriage is increased in women whose partners are over 35.[7]

The other finding is that the body of a man over 35 is less capable of seeking out and destroying damaged sperm, resulting in sperm with more DNA damage. This means that either there is less chance of getting pregnant or it could lead to a miscarriage or birth defects. It is estimated that 'older' fathers can be up to five times more likely to have children with birth defects. They have also been found to be six times more likely to have autistic children.[8]

We know that a high level of DNA fragmentation in sperm can be a cause of male infertility, increasing with age. But DNA fragmentation can only be detected using a special test on sperm – not a normal semen analysis . A high level could well be a crucial factor in unexplained infertility, low fertilisation rates in IVF, poor embryo quality, implantation failure after IVF and recurrent miscarriage. Men over the age of 35–40 should also be tested for DNA fragmentation of sperm even if they have had children before because research has shown that couples are much more likely to achieve a successful pregnancy either naturally or through assisted conception if DNA fragmentation is less than 30 per cent. The best-case scenario is less than 15 per cent indicating no problems with fertility, 15–30 per cent are of medium quality and over 30 per cent can affect fertility. (See page 218 for how to organise this test).

So is it possible to reduce a high level of DNA fragmentation?

DNA fragmentation can be caused by exposure to toxins, such as smoking or chemicals from either the environment or from the diet. Therefore, by making diet and lifestyle changes it is possible to reduce a high level of DNA fragmentation.

It takes almost three months for sperm to be produced so if a toxin hits the sperm during that period of development then DNA damage can happen. It is particularly important then for men to eliminate smoking, alcohol, hot baths, saunas and additives, preservatives and artificial sweeteners in foods when trying to conceive anyway, but is even more important when aiming to reduce a high DNA fragmentation level. Their diet should be as healthy as possible with good levels of fruit and vegetables and organic food should be used for two reasons: it is more likely that the food will contain higher levels of valuable minerals like zinc and selenium but, more crucially with respect to DNA fragmentation, eating organic will reduce exposure to toxins in the form of pesticides and herbicides.

Another important factor in DNA fragmentation is body weight. We know that when BMI (Body Mass Index) is over 25 (classed as overweight) fragmentation rises and it becomes even more of a problem when the BMI is over 30 (classed as obese).

Another way to help lower sperm fragmentation is to increase antioxidant intake. Antioxidants are powerful substances that are known to guard against DNA damage by protecting the body from toxins and pollutants. Selenium, zinc, vitamins A, C and E are all antioxidants and are generally found in brightly coloured fruit and vegetables (carrots, pumpkins, broccoli, berries, beetroot and tomatoes, for example). They are also in oily fish, nuts and seeds.

If your partner has been told he has a high DNA sperm fragmentation I would also recommend taking these nutrients in supplement form for quicker results. One study in 2005 looked at men with more than 15 per cent DNA fragmentation. They were given 1000mg vitamin C and 1000mg vitamin E for two months following one failed ICSI attempt. Seventy-six per cent of the men had a decrease in their percentage of DNA fragmentation and a second ICSI was performed. There was a staggering difference in the number of pregnancies (48.2 per cent compared to 6.9 per cent) on this second ICSI treatment and implantation rates went from 2.2 per cent to 19.6 per cent.[9]

Manganese (see page 84) is also important as it helps to activate an enzyme called superoxide dismutase (SOD). SOD protects the mitochondria (microscopic structures containing genetic material found in cells) from free radical attack. Interestingly, we all know that folic acid is important for women when trying to conceive but it is also crucial for men. It is needed for cell replication and growth and also helps with the healthy synthesis of DNA so it is an important supplement for men to take when reducing high fragmentation levels.[10] Because they are so important, men should take manganese and folic acid as supplements but they can be included in their multivitamin and mineral supplement and need not be taken separately.

So although age is important in male fertility it is not the only factor affecting sperm quality. Men produce sperm all their lives so it is possible to improve its quality and quantity through healthy lifestyle and nutritional changes.

Finally, it's not widely known that the egg has the ability to overcome any defects in the sperm. But as the eggs get older, this ability diminishes. So if you are over 35 it really is critical that your partner does all he can to make his sperm as healthy as possible.

(See also Step 4, pages 91–109, for more information on environmental and occupational hazards that can affect male fertility.)

IF YOU SMOKE – QUIT

If either you or your partner (see below) is a smoker my advice to you is simple: you need to quit! According to a report in February 2004 by the British Medical Association (BMA) smoking damages the reproductive system for both men and women.

Many studies have confirmed that women who do not smoke are twice as likely to get pregnant as women who do.[11] At the moment it is not entirely clear how smoking damages fertility but it could have a negative effect on egg quality by making them age prematurely; a condition known as accelerated atresia.[12]

Smoking also affects hormone balance by making the levels of FSH (follicle-stimulating hormone – see page 46) significantly higher than they should be, again making your eggs old before their time. It can even bring on irregular periods and an early menopause[13] by lowering oestrogen levels to those more typically seen in a menopausal woman. This is especially significant if you are over the age of 35 and are already racing against time.

Smoking depletes the level of vitamin C in your bloodstream and, as we saw in Step 1 (see page 25), good levels of antioxidants are crucial for improving egg quality. Women who smoke usually have high levels of a toxic metal called cadmium which can stop the utilisation of zinc, a mineral that is especially important for the reproductive system. Also, if you smoke, there is an undoubted and proven increased risk of miscarriage.[14] It is estimated that smoking is responsible for up to 5,000 miscarriages a year and that women who smoke just one cigarette a day reduce their chances of becoming pregnant and increase the likelihood of miscarriage.

In short, the more you smoke, the less likely you are to conceive. In fact, women whose mothers smoked during their pregnancy are less likely to conceive compared with those whose mothers were non-smokers. Passive smoking is also dangerous. Research shows that it can increase the risk of a miscarriage.[15]

IF YOUR PARTNER SMOKES

Apart from affecting erectile function, smoking can also directly impact on sperm in terms of count, motility and morphology (whether the sperm are a normal shape or not). In general, it has been shown that men with low sperm counts and/or low motility and/or abnormal sperm have lower vitamin C levels than men with normal semen analyses.[16]

Smoking also has a negative effect on the head of the sperm making it harder to fertilise an egg.[17] Researchers from the University of Buffalo, USA, studied men who had smoked at least four cigarettes a day for more than two years and compared them with non-smokers. They placed half of the zona pellucida – the shell surrounding the egg – with smokers' sperm and the other half with non-smokers'. After several hours they looked to see how many of the sperm were attached tightly and found that the sperm of two thirds of the smokers had failed the test. Those who did fail were 75 per cent less fertile than non-smokers. It is thought that nicotine overloads the receptors on sperm, affecting their ability to bind to the egg.

Smoking can also cause DNA damage to sperm and a study published in the *British Journal of Cancer* showed that men who smoke run the risk of fathering children who develop cancers such as leukaemia and brain tumours, even when their partner does not smoke.[18] One in seven childhood cancers could be due to the father's smoking habits. Just 1–9 cigarettes a day increased the risk by 3 per cent, 10–20 by 31 per cent and 20 or more by 42 per cent. Given the theory that chemicals in tobacco smoke can damage the DNA in sperm, it's easy to see that changes in DNA in the sperm could lead to a possible increase in the miscarriage rate. That is why a test for DNA damage can be so useful.

But smoking can bring other problems when trying to conceive because it can lead to impotence. Cigarette smoking causes damage to the blood vessels that supply the penis, altering blood flow and affecting circulation. One medical study was aptly called, 'A cigarette after sex, or instead of it'.[19]

SMOKING AND FERTILITY TREATMENT

Although there isn't an official anti-smoking policy from the Human Fertilisation and Embryology Authority (HFEA), they strongly advise against it when couples are undergoing fertility treatment. And it's not unheard of for individual fertility clinics or specialists to refuse fertility treatment if their clients are heavy smokers.

We know that smoking reduces the chances of success for IUI, IVF and ICSI.[20] One study showed that if couples smoke during the IVF cycle the number of eggs retrieved is decreased by 40 per cent and 46 per cent if just the man smokes during the cycle. Also, the overall success rate of the IVF was 44 per cent for non-smokers and 24 per cent for smokers.[21] Dutch scientists have also confirmed that smoking has a 'devastating' effect on the success of IVF treatment. In women with unexplained infertility, the live birth rate for smokers was 13 per cent compared with 20 per cent for non-smokers. Smokers were also more likely to miscarry.[22]

The good news is that within a year of stopping smoking ex-smokers took no longer to conceive than women who had never smoked. [23]

Finally, giving up smoking now can also make a difference to the next generation. Scientists have discovered that a child whose grandmother smoked during pregnancy has nearly double the chance of developing asthma even if their mother does not smoke. It is thought that the toxic chemicals in tobacco smoke can damage the baby girl's egg or even cause genetic changes.[24] Also research has shown that girls who didn't smoke but whose mothers did suffer a significantly increased risk of miscarriage.[25]

HOW SMOKING COULD AFFECT YOUR BABY-TO-BE

So smoking can make your eggs age faster, reduce your chances of conceiving and of having successful fertility treatment; the other problem is that if you are smoking and trying to conceive you are going to be two weeks pregnant before you know you are, so you need to quit before you even start trying to conceive. Tobacco smoke contains more than 4,000 compounds that pass directly into the baby's blood supply and these chemicals have different effects on the developing baby.

No fewer than 45 studies have confirmed that smoking is a major cause of low birth weight. Lack of oxygen to the developing baby (called foetal hypoxia) from cigarette smoking during pregnancy also leads to a higher risk of prematurity and congenital abnormalities.[26] Pregnant women who smoke 30 cigarettes a day have a 33 per cent likelihood of having a premature baby, compared to only 6 per cent of non-smoking mothers. Studies have found that smokers (both male and female) are more likely to have children with all types of congenital malformations – in particular, cleft palate, harelip, squints and deafness. Even if you don't smoke, having a partner who smokes over ten cigarettes a day can increase your risk of having a baby with congenital abnormalities (birth defects) by two and a half times.

The evidence is overwhelming that smoking should be avoided if you're trying to get pregnant, during pregnancy and breastfeeding and beyond. If your partner insists on smoking, he should not smoke in the house or when you are with him. Only 15 per cent of the smoke from a cigarette is inhaled – the remainder goes into the air and will be inhaled by those near to the smoker. Children of parents who smoke inhale amounts of nicotine equivalent to smoking 60 to 150 cigarettes a year. This results in an increased risk of asthma, chest, ear, nose and throat infections. It is estimated that 50 children a day are admitted to hospital due to the effects of passive smoking.[27]

ALCOHOL

Like smoking, alcohol can interfere with your fertility. Research has shown that women who drink heavily stop ovulating and menstruating and take longer to conceive. Alcohol intake has even been found to be a predictor for infertility in women.

A study in Denmark followed over 7,000 women who had never been pregnant over nearly five years and asked about their alcohol intake, smoking and any previous gynaecological problems. The researchers found that alcohol intake was a significant predictor for infertility among women above the age of 30.[28] In that age group, women who drank seven or more alcoholic drinks a week were twice as likely not to conceive as those women who drank less than one.

A study in the *British Medical Journal* in 1998 states categorically, that women should avoid alcohol when trying to conceive; women drinking 5 units or less a week were twice as likely to conceive within six months as women drinking 10 or more.[29] In 2004 another study followed thousands of women for 18 years and concluded that it was 'Important for the female partner in an infertile couple to limit alcohol intake or to not drink at all.'[30]

It appears that alcohol may prevent enough progesterone – one of the major players in ensuring a pregnancy stays put – from being produced by the egg capsule (corpus luteum). Even moderate drinking is linked to an increased risk of infertility in some women.[31] In one preliminary study there was a greater than 50 per cent reduction in the probability of conception in the menstrual cycle of women who drank alcohol.

We also now know that even small amounts of alcohol during pregnancy can slow down the unborn baby's growth with fears that it may later lead to behavioural problems and learning difficulties. Significant effects have been found with as little as one drink a day. This means that *there is no safe level in pregnancy.*

Complete abstinence for expectant mothers has been advocated for many years now in the USA, Canada, Australia, New Zealand and France. The very latest UK government policy states that for women who are over three months pregnant it is all right to drink one glass of wine a day. Given all the considerable scientific evidence though, my advice is not to drink any alcohol at all once pregnant.

It is estimated that one in 100 babies born in the UK is affected by the mother's drinking, suffering from hyperactivity and learning difficulties at one end of the spectrum to brain damage and deafness at the other. Full blown Foetal Alcohol Syndrome causes brain damage, mental retardation, flattened features, short stature, low birth weight and heart and kidney abnormalities. But a milder form called Foetal Alcohol Spectrum Disorder (FASD) can cause more subtle problems such as poor co-ordination and attention deficit disorder (ADD). The average IQ of a child with FASD is 20–80 points lower than the national average.

Some women say to me that they will stop smoking and/or drinking once they know they are pregnant. The irony is that it may be just those factors that are making it so hard for them to get pregnant in the first place. Furthermore, a woman is going to be pregnant for two weeks before she knows she is and it is in those first weeks that the highest rate of cell division for the developing baby takes place. Having a toxin, like alcohol, going into the body at that crucial time is not good and can have a huge impact on the health of the developing baby and all its structures and organs.

YOUR PARTNER AND ALCOHOL

It's not just you who needs to cut down – your partner does too. Alcohol can cause abnormalities in the head of the sperm which is critical for fertilisation of the egg.[32]

Also, alcohol reduces the level of vital sperm-making hormones, so a man can wipe out his sperm count for several months after a drinking session. Because of this it makes sense for a man to stop drinking for at least three months before trying to get his partner pregnant.

EXERCISE

Becoming as healthy and as fertile as you can involves both you and your partner exercising regularly.

For women who want to get pregnant exercise is particularly beneficial. Not only can it kick-start weight loss but it has also been proven to help insulin and glucose control, which in turn means balanced blood sugar levels, which are important for hormonal balance and fertility (see pages 33–34).[33] Exercise can also help you feel good about yourself. When you feel good, you'll be less inclined to eat unhealthy foods and will feel more positive towards your fertility-boosting plan; you're also likely to want to have sex more often because you will be happier with your body.[34]

You don't have to be fit to be fertile but it sure can help. A recent study showed that an improvement in fitness was as effective as weight reduction in boosting fertility.[35] Regular exercise can regulate your hormones and menstrual cycle in a beneficial way by helping you reach a healthy body weight and keeping stress levels down, therefore encouraging regular ovulation. Don't overdo it though. Training for more than 15 hours a week will have the opposite effect and inhibit ovulation. Women who exercise to the extreme, such as gymnasts and dancers and athletes, can lose their menstrual cycle because of the reduction in body weight.[36]

A good, balanced exercise programme provides three important benefits: stamina, strength and flexibility. A woman needs all three to lift and carry a baby, run after a small child, and cope with the day-to-day stresses of motherhood. Plus, getting in shape at least three months before you conceive may make it easier to maintain an active lifestyle during pregnancy and actually enjoy those nine months. Strengthening your back muscles now, for example, can stave off lower-back pain later. And aerobic exercise can improve your mood and energy levels, not to mention help you achieve a healthy pre-pregnancy weight.

HOW MUCH EXERCISE?

All you need is at least 30 minutes of moderate-intensity physical activity over and above your usual activity at work or home on most days of the week. If you can't set aside one block of time, or your fitness levels aren't there yet, try shorter sessions – say three ten-minute walks, for example. That's just as beneficial. If, of course, you can do more, go for it and extend your daily workout to 60 minutes. Don't overdo it though, as that can have a negative effect on your health and well-being! On top of any exercise, try to boost your daily activity levels further by doing things like getting off the bus a few stops earlier and walking, taking the stairs instead of the lift, walking to the shops and so on. When it comes to exercise every little helps.

YOUR DAILY ROUTINE

Once you've made the decision to exercise regularly the next thing you need to know is what goals you should be setting. A good exercise routine that you can repeat daily or three to five times a week at least starts with five to ten minutes of gentle warm-up, such as walking at a moderate pace, to raise your body temperature and increase your heart rate.

This is followed by a period of continuous moderate-paced aerobic conditioning. Aim for 20 to 30 minutes of continuous exercise that works the large muscles of the body and elevates your breathing and heart rate. Fast walking is ideal or you may prefer jogging, swimming or an exercise class.

The key is to give your muscles a good workout and get your heart pumping. As you increase the intensity of your workout your muscles need more oxygen and your heart beats faster. For weight loss you need to get your heart rate up to 60 to 75 per cent of its maximum capacity (220 minus your age) for around 20 to 45 minutes. If you feel slightly out of breath but not so much that you can't carry on a conversation you know you are exercising at the right rate. A cool-down should follow your aerobic workout.

AEROBIC EXERCISE SUGGESTIONS

Any activity that gets you slightly out of breath is aerobic. Try to choose something you enjoy and will want to continue. The following aerobic exercises are well suited to women in the pre-conception period as they give you a great workout with the minimum of fuss and stress. Aim for around 30 minutes of continuous exercise every day or every other day. If you're a beginner, start with ten minutes and gradually build to 30 minutes over a period of three to four months.

Walking

When you begin your walking programme, start slowly, maybe with a five-minute stroll. Each time you walk, increase your intensity by walking faster and for longer until you walk for 20 or 30 minutes. You can also add light hand weights while emphasising arm movements. If you don't want to walk outside you can try using a treadmill.

Swimming

Swimming is a great way to exercise as it works every muscle in the body with the minimum of stress. If you enjoy swimming, as with walking, start by going to the pool twice a week for a gentle 15-minute swim. Gradually increase the length of your swim, and your work rate while in the water, building up to about 30 minutes a day, or 45 minutes twice a week. You might also want to try some aqua aerobic classes. Because of the way the water supports your body as you exercise it removes the stress factor and conditions your muscles with the minimum of discomfort.

Cycling/cycle-machine or jogging

As with walking or swimming, start with a short, easy routine, say 10–15 minutes a day, gradually working up to about 30 minutes a day. Gradually increase your work rate, without ever straining yourself. If you are jogging, you should invest in a good pair of running shoes that offer cushioned support.

Trampoline jogging

Gently jogging on a small trampoline can be a good aerobic workout. Try to keep going for 20 to 30 minutes. You can buy small, inexpensive trampolines from most sports shops.

Dancing

You can join a class, go to a disco or simply put on your favourite music at home and dance. Dancing isn't just fun it's a great way to exercise and release tension.

Be careful of any high-impact aerobics in the second half of the cycle just in case you are pregnant.

TONING AND STRETCHING

You also need to include some muscle-strengthening activities into your routine around two or three times a week – building up better muscle tone not only makes you look more streamlined but also boosts your metabolism because muscles burn more calories than fat.

Walking and cycling are good weight-bearing endurance exercises but strength training is even better. The aim is not to become muscle bound – you only need to do a few sets of exercises like press-ups (to work your upper body) and squats (to work your lower body). Fitness clubs offer instruction and weights and weight machines but if you can't face the gym you can work out at home with some light dumb-bells or heavy books/cans. An instructional video can also help. To get the most out of weight training you need to take the time to know how to perform the exercises with correct technique.

In addition to this you need to build in a daily routine that stretches your muscles and puts your joints through the full range of motion. The best time to stretch is when your muscles are warmed up after your aerobic workout. Allow about 10 minutes for stretching. Stretching your muscles keeps you flexible. It also lengthens your muscles and improves posture. T'ai chi and yoga are great ways to stretch.

HOW FIT ARE YOU?

Test yourself:

~ Can you walk briskly for ten minutes without feeling exhausted?

~ Can you walk up a flight of stairs without losing your breath?

~ Sit quietly and check your resting pulse rate. Find your pulse where your wrist joins your hand, just below the thumb and about 1cm from the edge of your wrists. Count the beats for 20 seconds then multiply by three. If the results are under 70 you are pretty fit, 80–100 is ok (-ish!), over 100 is not good and is a sign that you need to get fit.

SOME TIPS TO GET YOU GOING

Getting started with an exercise routine can be the biggest hurdle. The following tips will help get you going:

~ Choose an activity you enjoy so you can maintain a positive attitude – anything from dancing or skipping to rambling. Studies show that exercise dropouts often punish themselves with routines they don't enjoy. If you know you hate the gym, don't go.

~ Vary your exercise and activity routine, so you don't get bored.

~ Doing housework may not be the most fun, but it does get you moving! So do gardening and walking the dog.

~ Don't let the cold weather keep you on the sofa! You can still find activities to do in the winter like exercising to a workout video or joining a sports club. Or get a head start on your spring cleaning by choosing active indoor chores like window washing or reorganising cupboards.

~ Exercise with a friend or family member. It's tougher to break the commitment to exercise when you know someone else will be working out with you.

~ Make exercise into a social occasion – have lunch or dinner after you and a friend work out.

~ Read fitness books or magazines to inspire you.

~ Set specific, short-term fitness goals, and reward yourself when you achieve them.

~ Make your activity a regular part of your day, so – like healthy eating – it becomes a habit.

SLEEP

Not getting enough quality sleep makes it harder to handle stress and affects quality of life, according to a poll by the US National Sleep foundation. In addition to raising stress hormones which can trigger unwanted weight gain and fatigue, research shows that sleep deprivation results in hormonal imbalance, therefore increasing the risk of infertility.[37]

A good night's sleep is one of the best tonics you can have but it's important to realise that quality, not quantity, is the key. A recent study at Brigham and Women's Hospital in Boston, USA, showed that a good night's sleep makes you feel happier and more relaxed, but under six hours or over ten can make you feel irritable. Seven to eight hours seems ample for most people, but six hours of good-quality sleep beats a restless nine hours.

To encourage a good night's sleep:
~ avoid exercising at least two hours before you go to sleep
~ try to stick to a regular bedtime, preferably before midnight, and a regular waking time
~ make sure you keep fresh air circulating in your bedroom; the brain's sleep centre works better with oxygen
~ make sure your bedroom isn't too noisy, light, untidy, hot or cold
~ try a warm bath, perhaps with a few drops of lavender oil as this can have a sedative quality
~ use simple relaxation techniques before you go to sleep, such as gentle stretching or meditation
~ try valerian – it is classed as a sedative in herbal medicine; passionflower (or passiflora) is also good and can be used together with valerian for maximum effect
~ drink a cup of hot chamomile tea before bed.

TIME FOR SEX

Ironically, a number of couples seeking fertility treatment get so hung up on watching their weight or taking fertility-boosting supplements that they forget the most important part of baby-making: having sex.

To maximise your chances of pregnancy you should enjoy as much sex as possible, or at least two times a week. Lots of sex will help normalise your cycle and help your partner too, as the idea that abstaining from sex for up to a week so they save up sperm isn't helpful. Abstaining *will* stack up larger volumes of sperm but at the same time it will reduce its quality so that it's less likely to make you pregnant.[38]

It is better to have sex every alternate night than every night as this helps to build up good-quality sperm. When a man goes for a semen analysis, he is asked to abstain for at least three days as that is a good space of time (albeit a bit too long when you are trying to conceive) but not longer than seven because the quality diminishes after that.

As you'll see in Step 6, although timing is important to maximise your chances of getting pregnant you shouldn't become obsessed with the idea of timetable sex. In fact, your body may well help you to feel more sexy at the right times, anyway; some researchers believe that, like many animals, a desire for mating in humans is when a female ovulates. Many women say that not only do they feel sexier when they are ovulating but their partners feel more sexually stimulated at that time too. So let nature take its course and have sex when you want to – you're more likely to enjoy it then, too, which, in itself can bring about fertility benefits.

THE IMPORTANCE OF ORGASM

Two British biologists, Robin Baker and Mark Bellis, investigated the 'upsuck hypothesis' and discovered that when a woman climaxes any time between a minute before to 45 minutes after her lover ejaculates, she retains significantly more sperm than she does after non-orgasmic sex. In addition, their research results indicated that the strong muscular contractions associated with orgasm create a partial vacuum, which help to suck the sperm from the vagina to the cervix, where it's in a better position to reach an egg.

Evolutionary psychologists are suggesting that in the past orgasm could have served a purpose – unconsciously – in favouring the man that a woman wants to father her child. So the woman would have an orgasm with one man who she would like to have children with and not another.[39]

But it is important to remember that a woman does not need to have an orgasm in order to conceive. So do not beat yourself up if you do not have one every time you have intercourse.

SATISFYING SEX

Research[40] appears to suggest that women who have regular satisfying sex, with intercourse at least once a week, have more regular menstrual cycles and fewer fertility problems than those who don't. In addition, a satisfying sex life can be a wonderful way to reduce stress and therefore encourage fertility because, like exercise, it boosts the production of feel-good hormones.

A loving, caring, emotionally supportive relationship can also have a positive effect on your fertility. Women can spontaneously ovulate when they fall in love and there is growing evidence that when you feel happy and secure and loved and have a fulfilling sex life, fertility can prosper. That isn't to say that being single, or having an argument or break-up will affect your fertility, or that a bad relationship can't produce a baby, but if your love life is chronically stressful this could well be contributing to any fertility problems.

JUST TOO TIRED!

It's all very well knowing that you should be enjoying regular, satisfying sex, but what if you're too stressed and too tired?

A new condition called TINS is a real threat to fertility rates. It stands for Two Incomes No Sex. According to research by a British organisation called the Chartered Institute of Personal Development, over half the people they interviewed said their sex lives were suffering because of the long hours they spent at work.

If you're finding it hard to get in the mood or just feel too tired, the following recommendations might help to kick-start your libido:

~ Eat healthily according to the fertility-boosting diet guidelines (see pages 14–33) as fatigue is a symptom of nutritional deficiency. And it's not an old wives' tale that oysters help with sex drive – it is because they are high in zinc and zinc is good for libido in both partners! The B vitamins and selenium are crucial too.
~ Exercise helps by boosting your mood and body image.
~ Check your stress levels. In general, stress dampens libido. Deal with commonplace stress by following the de-stressing tips on page 65.
~ Depression can be a major inhibitor of sexual desire. Try to understand why you are feeling low, so that you act appropriately when low feelings hit you. If you feel you can't cope alone, reach out for the support of family and friends or see your doctor for a referral to a counsellor or therapist.
~ Get a good night's sleep (see page 58). When you are tired the libido is usually the first thing to go. The bottom line is that you can survive without sex but you can't survive without sleep.
~ Most sex therapists agree that sex begins in the head – in a way it's an idea that overtakes you and which your body then follows. So setting the mood can really help – music, low lighting, a candlelit bath, or your favourite romantic or raunchy film.
~ If you haven't felt sexy for a while, touching yourself can also be a way to reconnect with your body as a sensual, sexual pleasure. Once you're back in touch with your own desires it can be easier and less daunting to connect with your partner's.
~ Make time for romance. However busy you are, try to make sure that you have some

'couple time' where you can unwind together and talk about your day. And plan regular meals out, cinema trips or weekend breaks so that the two of you get some special time together away from the hustle and bustle of everyday life.

Communicate
Relationship troubles can also contribute to a loss of sexual desire. If you don't feel listened to, respected or important it is natural to respond with resentment and that, in turn, can dampen libido. It's important to open the lines of communication with your partner so that anger can be expressed in places other than the bedroom. If the problem is severe (such as infidelity) you may want to go to a relationship counsellor.

If you find the idea of sex unappealing or uncomfortable, talk to a sex therapist to discuss your health, your upbringing, your circumstances, any body image issues you may have and your relationship so that you can find ways to give yourself permission to satisfy your sexual needs. You may want to do this alone or you may find that it is more productive to talk to a sex therapist with your partner.

Herbs
There are numerous herbal treatments which are thought to help put sexual desire and drive back into your life and these include American ginseng, agnus castus and damiana. It's important to take herbs with professional advice though, as remember you are going to be two weeks pregnant before you know you are.
Note: it is important that if you are having any kind of fertility treatment with drugs you should stop taking herbs but keep taking nutritional supplements.

Aromatherapy
Aromatherapists believe that certain scents, such as jasmine, rose and sandalwood can have an aphrodisiac effect. Smell works through association too. Returning to a perfume you used to wear when you first met your partner may rekindle the passion. Other studies show that the scent of popcorn and vanilla can be a real turn-on for both men and women. (See also pages 75–76.)

TRYING TOO HARD?
You've probably heard stories of couples who tried really hard to get pregnant and only conceived once they had given up. However, it's only when 'trying' turns from a natural, loving desire to have a baby into an anxiety-, fear- and worry-filled pursuit that there can be problems. If you feel calm and confident about your sexuality and are in a loving and healthy relationship there is no such thing as 'trying too hard' to have a

baby. So make diet and lifestyle changes (see pages 14 and 33) but above all, stay calm and enjoy your sex life. (See also Common Fertility Misconceptions, page 137).

OVER-THE-COUNTER DRUGS

There are certain medications that can interfere with your fertility or that of your partner and it is important that you are aware of their potential effects. For example, it is thought that medications such as the antihistamine cimetidine and sulphasalazine (used to treat ulcerative colitis) and long-term daily use of some antibiotics and androgen injections can affect semen quality and cause an extremely low sperm count. Usually these negative side effects will be reversed within three months of stopping the medication, but some medications, such as beta-blockers and psychotropic drugs may lead to impotence.[41]

Steroids such as cortisone and prednisone, which are used to treat conditions such as asthma and lupus, can prevent your pituitary gland from producing enough follicle-stimulating hormone (FSH) and luteinising hormone (LH) for normal ovulation to occur, but only if you take the medications in high doses. Some older antihypertensive medications which are used to control blood pressure can raise your prolactin levels and also interfere with ovulation. However, most modern antidepressants (selective serotonin reuptake inhibitors or SSRIs) do not have a negative affect on ovulation or fertility.

Almost any drug that targets the central nervous system – tranquillisers, painkillers or seizure-prevention medications can affect prolactin and/or the ability of the pituitary gland to promote ovulation. Even ordinary over-the-counter drugs, such as paracetamol and ibuprofen, can inhibit the production of prostaglandins which are essential for the healthy development of the foetus. Taking analgesics or painkillers – the kind you buy at the chemist and supermarket – has also been to shown to increase the risk of miscarriage[42] and paracetamol has been linked to causing mutations in human cells.[43] Many women take thyroid medication, but if too much or too little is prescribed, it can also affect ovulation.

Aspirin use, even moderate (one or two a week), has been shown to cause a significant decrease in sperm motility.[44] Although preliminary research suggests that low-dose aspirin may actually have a beneficial effect for women, the Royal College of Obstetrics and Gynaecology still advises women concerned about their fertility to check with their doctor before taking aspirin, paracetamol, ibuprofen or any kind of painkiller because they may increase the risk of miscarriage.

You should try to avoid taking any drugs while pregnant and if you are taking any sleeping pills, tranquillisers or painkillers talk to your doctor about coming off them and finding other ways to deal with the problems. Different drugs affect different people in different ways. This may be to do with how efficient the liver is at making enzymes to break the drugs down and also to do with the mother's nutritional state because if she is poorly nourished she will tend to clear drugs out of her system more slowly.

If you are worried about the fertility effects of any drugs that you have taken, do seek advice from your doctor. When in doubt, if you need to take any over-the-counter or prescription drugs make sure you first discuss its impact on your fertility with your pharmacist or doctor.

STREET DRUGS

There is growing evidence that street drugs produce side effects that can damage fertility in both men[45] and women. But what if you use cocaine, marijuana, amphetamines, ecstasy or anabolic steroids casually? The advice is still to give up because even if these drugs haven't been directly linked to lowered fertility they have been shown to have other adverse health effects ranging from dehydration to depression and, in a few isolated cases, death.

Marijuana can lower a man's levels of FSH and LH, two hormones vital for sperm production. It can also lower his libido. The use of marijuana by the father-to-be has also been linked to cot death.[46] In women it can lead to irregular periods and lack of ovulation.[47]

Cocaine users will have a lower sperm count, poorly moving sperm and a high rate of abnormal sperm and heroin can cause a decrease in testosterone levels.[48] If taken together cocaine and heroin will make it harder for a woman to conceive and she is more likely to have a miscarriage, a stillbirth or a baby born with a malformation.[49]

As well as their adverse effects on fertility and libido these drugs can also affect the development and health of the growing baby. In animals marijuana has been linked to stillbirths and malformations[50] and women who use cocaine in pregnancy are more likely to miscarry or have a baby with a malformation.[51] Also babies born to mothers who have taken heroin and cocaine suffer withdrawal symptoms.

So the message is that street drugs need to be eliminated from your body at least four months before you try for a baby.

STRESS

If you're trying for a baby stress management is important because too much stress can trigger the release of the stress hormone cortisol. Too much cortisol in your bloodstream can interfere with your hormonal balance – in particular the output of sex hormones – and affect the functioning of the hypothalamus and the pituitary (the glands in the brain that regulate your appetite and emotions), as well as the hormones that tell your ovaries to release eggs.

It's not unusual for me to see women with irregular or absent periods and to learn that they are also going through some kind of stress or trauma. Studies show that extreme stress can interfere with and stop ovulation or play havoc with the delicate balance of hormones needed for healthy ovulation.[52] For example, losing a close family member can take its toll on fertility. And according to a recent study[53] stresses like separation, divorce, illness and a pressurised job all raised the likelihood of miscarriage, with those who felt relaxed and happy early in pregnancy being 60 per cent less likely to miscarry.

It's not just extreme stress either – everyday tension and experiences can all have an effect – even the prospect of a driving test can be enough to make you miss a period. This mechanism seems to be nature's way of preventing pregnancy at a time when a woman may find it hard to cope.

Stress also affect a man's hormone balance too[54] and some researchers suggest that stress causes infertility because it triggers the production of malformed eggs, or sperm or both. Pregnancies created by damaged sperm or egg tend to result in miscarriages so early that you may not even realise you are pregnant and think you are having a particularly heavy period.

Stress in men can also interfere with the hormones controlling sperm production. Research has shown that men under stress at work or home are more likely to have poor sperm quality.[55] One study of 157 men conducted by the University of California in 1997[56] showed that a very depressing experience, like the loss of a loved one, can temporarily reduce a man's sperm count. Other research shows that stress or unhappiness can lower sperm count and make remaining sperm move badly and even have cell abnormalities. Stress has also been shown to have an impact on the quality of sperm of men in couples undergoing the rollercoaster of stress that often goes hand in hand with IVF.[57]

Couples who have been trying for a baby without success often experience high levels of stress, especially if they need medical assistance and the longer it takes the more anxious they become and the more chance there is of stress inhibiting fertility. Some studies on animals and humans also show that if a woman becomes extremely anxious about getting pregnant she may release eggs that are not mature enough to be fertilised.[58]

Finally, higher than normal levels of stress hormone can lower libido in both men and women because they have a knock-on effect on the hormones that power sex drive

– oestrogen and testosterone. And not having enough sex or enjoying satisfying sex, as we saw earlier, may be a prime cause of infertility (see page 58).

Progressive fertility units such as the Beth Israel Hospital in Boston, USA, and Harvard Behavioral Medicine Program have been including stress reduction in their programmes for 15 years. 'Our experience at the Division Behavioral Medicine in the Beth Israel Deaconess Medical Center, and this is backed up by research,[59] is that women with long-term infertility may well increase their chances of conception when they reduce their levels of stress and depression,' says Alice Domar, director of the Mind/Body Institute at the centre.

The International Europe survey of 2000 has identified stressful work as a major factor in infertility.[60] It seems that high public contact jobs, and high-stress jobs such as being an air stewardess, teacher or nurse, increase the risk of miscarriage. There's more about occupational health risks in Step 4 (pages 91–109), but for now bear in mind that if you are feeling stressed for whatever reason – be it anxiety about your fertility, or worry about your job or upset because of troubles in your relationship – you may well find that this interferes with your health and fertility.

As I've highlighted throughout this book infertility is clearly a multi-faceted problem. This is why we are looking at every possibility, not only the physical and lifestyle aspects (like diet and exercise) but also the emotional and psychological ones, like stress and anxiety. Stress is a fact of life and you can't avoid it, but you can find ways to manage it and the stress-management tips below will help you to do just that. In fact, simply recognising that you are stressed or anxious can be an important step. Do bear in mind that any stress-management regime needs to begin with a healthy eating plan (Step 1) to ensure that your body remains fit and able to cope during stressful times.

TOP STRESS-MANAGEMENT TIPS

~ Take a good multivitamin and mineral supplement. The adrenal glands rely on vitamins C, B5 and B6, zinc and magnesium and these are rapidly depleted when you are under stress, so a good multivitamin and mineral every day makes sense, especially one that is designed for fertility (e.g. Fertility Plus for women).

~ Meditation is a great way to lower both physical and mental stress. To have a go at meditation by yourself find a quiet place where you won't be interrupted. Make sure you are comfortable, and then start to imagine each part of your body from your toes to your scalp relaxing, while mentally repeating a neutral thought (try a colour). When other thoughts break through the calm just let them come and go. After ten minutes open your eyes and sit quietly for a few moments before getting up. Researchers at the University of Dublin found that when women with high stress levels were given relaxation-training techniques their stress levels dropped to normal and their menstrual cycles returned to normal.

~ Massage can help. The sense of well-being you get from a massage can lower the amount of stress hormones, such as cortisol, circulating throughout your body. Either book a session with a qualified practitioner, or if you have time and think it would be fun, use a good book or a video to learn some simple techniques for yourself or with your partner.

~ Take up yoga. The UK's leading mental health charity, MIND, recommends yoga as the single most effective stress-buster. Yoga has been around for thousands of years and its benefits remain constant. The poses aim to bring your mind, body and breathing together to improve posture and physical health and bring a sense of calm.

~ Think about how you react to stress and identify people and situations that trigger it. You can't avoid every trigger but you don't have to invite them into your life. Use simple relaxation techniques to deal with short-term stress. For example, if you get tense when stuck in traffic, try simple techniques such as tensing your muscles hard and relaxing them, or deep breathing for a count of ten or daydreaming about a holiday. Other techniques include drinking calming herbal teas like chamomile, having a good laugh, chatting to a friend, reading a good book or listening to soothing music. Set aside ten or twenty minutes a day to relax, no matter what.

~ The regular exercise you're hopefully already doing as part of your fertility-boosting plan is also great for beating stress. Not only does it stimulate the body's pituitary gland to release tension and give you a natural high, it also tires you out so you sleep better, no matter how much your mind is racing. Research also shows that regular exercise makes you less tense and better able to cope with stress.

~ Try not to be a perfectionist. Let the dishes sit in the dishwasher a little longer, return that call tomorrow, wear clothes you feel comfortable in.

~ Learn to manage your time more effectively and each day won't seem such a struggle. Plan your day and prioritise what needs to be done. Tackle one task at a time and allow extra time for the unexpected.

~ Stress forces you to take shallow breaths that prevent your body from getting rid of tension in the way that a deep breath can. A large lung full of air centres and calms you. Most of us take tiny shallow breaths. Practise this breathing technique the next time you feel stressed: to a count of four breathe in through your nose, right down into your stomach, hold for one, and then push the breath out, again for a count of four.

EASING EMOTIONAL STRESS FOR FERTILITY

Emotional health is as important for your fertility as physical health. You've seen how your body is unlikely to ovulate if you aren't eating properly and, as we have seen, your reproductive hormones can stop working properly if you are unhappy or distressed.

Stresses that have been found to suppress ovulation and menstrual cycle function include low self-esteem, poor body image, negative or ambivalent feelings about a relationship and the prospect of motherhood. Research has also shown that in some cases women who don't ovulate can be more anxious and have lower self-esteem than those who do.[61]

Without a doubt the state of your mind and body are connected. (Why else do you always seem to get a cold when you are stressed?) And whether you are undergoing fertility treatment or not, anxiety about getting pregnant may be one of the biggest stresses you encounter on your fertility journey, with the constant 'Will it happen?' question going around inside your head.

As you've seen any kind of stress has a negative effect on fertility. The suggestions below should help but if you are finding that the stress of your fertility journey is destroying your quality of life and your relationships do talk to your doctor who can put you in touch with a counsellor to help you work through your feelings.

Don't put your life on hold

There's a temptation to put the rest of your life on 'hold' because you don't know what lies ahead. Should you plan to go on a holiday next month – what if you get pregnant? Should your husband accept a new job, even if it means a transfer to another city – you will then have to find a new doctor or clinic? It can be frustrating when you feel that not only are you not getting pregnant, but you also cannot get on with the rest of your life. You need to try to separate infertility from other important aspects of your life.

Don't become obsessive

Don't allow yourself to get so obsessed with your fertility that every other aspect of your life suffers, including your relationship. It has been heartbreaking in the clinic to see couples separate or divorce from the strains of fertility investigations and treatments. Remember it takes average couples around a year to get pregnant so take the pressure off yourself in terms of how fast you expect pregnancy to happen.

Stay positive, but realistic

Think positive, but be realistic. Stay optimistic about your chances of getting pregnant, but be aware that there is a chance you may not be able to conceive. By maintaining a practical mindset, you can help to make the best decisions about your fertility treatment for yourself and your partner, which is crucial in coping with infertility issues.

Maintain a positive self-image
Don't blame yourself for your infertility issues; it is very easy to fall into the trap of feeling guilty, angry or insecure when you're experiencing a fertility problem. You must remember that you are a worthy person irrespective of your fertility. Staying positive and reminding yourself that it is your fertility that is failing and not you will help you reframe the experience in a less negative light.

Keep your life as full as possible
While undergoing fertility testing and treatments can take up a lot of your time, try to cultivate some time for relaxing. Take up a class that's always interested you, such as dance or creative writing. Make Tuesday nights movie night and rent a favourite comedy to take your own and your partner's mind off things. This will help you unwind and keep a positive attitude towards getting pregnant.

Down time
Nurture yourself with relaxation techniques, such as deep breathing from the abdomen, not the chest; meditation; guided imagery or yoga. Or simply zone out and daydream every so often. Allow your mind to wander for five minutes every time you feel tense. Maybe use a favourite picture or holiday memory to help you daydream, or find places you know make you feel relaxed and spend some time there as often as you can, even if it's only ten minutes in the park at lunchtime.

BE MINDFUL Mindfulness is the technique of living in the here and now and enjoying the present moment. One of the peculiar effects of infertility is that it tends to be so totally absorbing. Your concentration is on the next step in your treatment, on what your ovulation kit will show next week, whether you dare to travel next month, did you have sex enough when you ovulated and so on. Soon there is no room in your mind for what is actually going on around you.

By being mindful – by concentrating on every aspect of what you are doing, such as the lunch you are eating, walking down a street, or completing a task – you are both relaxing and nurturing yourself. Your feelings of being stressed vanish as you focus on finding pleasure in the present moment.

THE DREADED 'ARE YOU PREGNANT YET'?

When you're trying to get pregnant you may find that the expectations of others can be very hard to deal with. If you do find yourself being asked the inevitable 'Are you pregnant?' question by thoughtless people you can either turn this into an opportunity for you to explain your situation more fully (to close friends) or you can discourage further discussion. Here are some typically painful questions or comments you may well encounter and for which you may want to be prepared:

~ So when are you going to start a family? You two aren't getting any younger!

~ When are you going to stop concentrating on your career and start a family?

~ Well, I guess we'll never be grandparents.

~ Oh, I have just the opposite problem – I get pregnant so easily; I think you just need to relax about it.

~ I wish you'd take one of my kids – they drive me crazy!

~ I hear they're having tremendous success with test-tube babies. Why don't you try it?

~ Any good news yet?

~ Things happen for a reason.

Be firm and pleasant and try not to get defensive. After all, just because a question is asked does not always mean it deserves an answer. With a smile, you can let people know that it's none of their business without being rude yourself.

TAKING CARE OF YOUR RELATIONSHIP

Infertility really tests a couple's relationship and shakes the foundation of a marriage. The good news is that the experience can ultimately strengthen the bond for most couples; but for some the emotional ups and downs of trying to conceive can result in a neglected marriage. Couples can easily forget the things that were good about their relationship in the first place.

One of your biggest challenges will be to see the situation through your partner's eyes. Infertility easily becomes the central focus of the woman's thoughts and feelings, whereas men tend to shift into problem-solving mode and be more optimistic from the start. The following recommendations may help you to use the experience to enhance your relationship:

~ Work as a team; no finger-pointing allowed. Create an environment of support as opposed to blame with your partner.

~ Plan playtime; don't let trying to conceive become a full-time job.

~ Separate baby-making from lovemaking. Use your imagination – designate different rooms for 'work' and 'play' and plan romance.

~ Build a support system. Neither of you can be everything for your partner. Seek balance through friends – and not just fellow trying-to-conceive buddies.

~ Identify individual coping styles under stress. Know and accept differences in how each of you deals with stress.

~ Allow breathing room in your relationship. You're not always in the same place emotionally. Give each other space and distance.

~ Communicate the positives. Don't let infertility be the sole topic of conversation. Discuss the good things, and set a 20-minute time limit on treatment talk.

~ Keep your sense of humour. Find the bright spots and laugh together.

~ Seek help before problems get too big. If your usual coping strategies aren't working or if you feel that your relationship has come to a grinding or sudden halt, don't wait to ask for help.

~ Take on tasks together in order to maintain a strong relationship. For example, if you require injections of fertility drugs, your partner can administer the shots for you.

~ Educate yourself about fertility problems. This will help you make informed choices about the type of fertility treatment you're undergoing and is an excellent way of coping with infertility. Also, because assisted reproductive technology changes so quickly, it can help you stay up-to-date with the latest forms of treatment.

~ Finally, establish limits on how long you're willing to try and how much you are willing to spend. Although it can be very difficult, choosing when to stop fertility treatments if you continue to have problems getting pregnant is a decision that any couple, along with their health care professional, might have to make. In fact, one third of couples who undergo fertility treatment are unable to have a biological child. Factors that may influence the amount of fertility treatment that you're prepared to undergo include your medical odds of getting pregnant, as well as the types of fertility treatment you are or are not willing to try.

HOW DO YOU DEAL WITH YOUR OWN EXPECTATIONS AND THOSE OF OTHERS AS YOU RIDE THE FERTILITY ROLLERCOASTER?

First of all admit to yourself that having problems getting pregnant is a difficult situation. Experiencing fertility problems is one of the hardest things that you will encounter in your life and acknowledgement of this is an important first step in coping. Realise that it is very normal to feel angry, stressed or sad about not getting pregnant easily. Confronting your emotions and accepting them will help you to move on with the process of getting pregnant.

Second, avoid people and situations that make you uneasy. If you are faced with something about which you feel uncomfortable, such as receiving yet another baby shower invite, don't feel you have to accept. Politely decline and send a gift; you may even purchase it online so as not to have to make a trip to a baby store. Don't feel guilty about this; acknowledge that it is emotionally upsetting and that sometimes you need to act in your own best interests.

Third, find people you can trust and with whom you want to share your emotions, feelings and stresses. Obviously you will rely heavily on your partner for support and back-up and he or she will know very well what you are going through. But forming a network that extends beyond your partner is also important. Talking to loved ones, friends and colleagues and explaining the frustrations you are going through can really help. People aren't mind-readers; unless you explain to them what is going on they can't help or support you. However, this isn't always an option – your family and friends may live too far away, you may not feel comfortable confiding in them or they may all have children and you feel the odd one out. If you have no one to talk to about your feelings it is time to contact a counsellor, or join a support group made up of couples trying to get pregnant, where you can discuss your feelings openly and learn about other people's experiences.

It can also be hard to know whether to tell work colleagues or not. If you tell them they may jump to the wrong conclusions and put your career on hold, thinking that you may get pregnant at any moment, not to mention the inevitable, 'Are you pregnant yet?' questions. But if you don't tell them what are you going to say every time you need to take time off for tests and appointments? If you don't tell anyone you could end up even more stressed having to invent reasons for your absences.

The important thing is to get beyond feeling that you need to explain yourself to everyone and to spend more time managing your condition and looking after yourself instead. The stressful nature of trying for a baby with or without fertility treatment is now recognised by experts the world over. Having a good cry can help you to let go of pent-up emotional stress, as can talking to your partner or other women with fertility problems. But learning how to manage feelings of stress and tension by taking your mind off things and staying positive so you don't get so many bad days is better still.

GIVE YOURSELF TIME

Research has shown that changing your diet and lifestyle and finding ways to manage stress can help you to conceive faster naturally and if not, you will in any case be in the best of health, ready for assisted conception, if you choose to go down that route.

The diet and lifestyle guidelines in Steps 1 and 2 are a lot to take in all in one go – so don't expect to be able to make the changes overnight. Ideally, you should be giving yourself a few weeks to put everything in place and to give yourself and your partner a chance to get used to following these guidelines, so that they become second nature. These are not 'miracle' cures that will mean you get pregnant overnight. What I do know, however, is that many women who have come to me with fertility problems have got pregnant after getting their diets, emotions and lifestyles into shape. So take a deep breath and be patient – stick to the plan and you might be amazed by how dramatic the results are.

INVESTIGATING COMPLEMENTARY THERAPIES

In the great majority of cases diet, lifestyle and supplementation are the most important factors in boosting fertility. If, however, you feel you want to give yourself some extra help you may want to try a complementary therapy that appeals to you and that you can afford.

In my practice I have had most success combining diet and lifestyle change with herbs but there's enough anecdotal evidence (and in some cases good scientific research) to suggest that the complementary therapies outlined below can maximise your chances of conceiving either with or without medical help.

Like orthodox medicine, complementary medicine doesn't have all the answers but it can have a great deal to offer because it looks at you holistically. This means it takes everything about you into consideration: your state of mind, your job, your health, and so on instead of focusing on a particular symptom, such as irregular periods. Perhaps the greatest benefit of the following complementary therapies is that they can all help you to deal with stress to some extent which is an important aspect of any fertility treatment (see pages 63–72).

HERBAL MEDICINE

Herbal medicine is the use of medicine made from plants (see page 87). Herbs have been traditionally used as fertility enhancers for centuries in many parts of the world. The use of agnus castus as a fertility herb has shown a prolific rise in Western countries and seems to be leading the field among herbs in this respect (see page 87).

However, other herbal remedies have great potential to relieve stress and encourage relaxation and therefore boost fertility. These include passionflower, chamomile and wild oat. Passionflower is considered one of the best tranquillising herbs because it is non-addictive and allows you to wake feeling fresh rather than bleary-eyed the next morning when it is taken to enhance sleep. Chamomile is a gentle and trusted relaxant of the nervous system and a popular and safe remedy for stress-related problems, anxiety, tension and insomnia. Wild oat or avena sativa is used especially for fatigue, stress, depression and anxiety.

ACUPUNCTURE

Acupuncture is a traditional Chinese medicine technique that uses hair-thin needles to treat pain, allergies and nausea. It is also showing promise as a treatment for female infertility.

The technique is based on the theory that vital energy (or 'qi', pronounced 'chi') flows through the body along certain pathways and practitioners try to balance this energy and restore health by stimulating specific points along the pathways with thin needles. Traditional acupuncturists treat the whole person rather than a disease and therefore attempt to get to the root cause of the problem rather than treating its symptoms. Like other holistic practitioners, they will consider all lifestyle and environmental factors before commencing treatment for infertility.

Although it has been a staple of Chinese medicine for some 5,000 years, acupuncture has gained greater acceptance in the medical community only in the past few decades.

Researchers from New York's Weill Cornell Medical Center recently reviewed existing studies and found that acupuncture helps to:

~ reduce stress hormones that interfere with ovulation

~ normalise hormones that regulate ovulation so an egg is released

~ increase blood flow to the uterus, improving the chances of a fertilised egg implanting

~ improve ovulation cycles in women with polycystic ovary syndrome (PCOS), which makes getting pregnant difficult; many women with PCOS seem to find it helpful in kick-starting absent periods or regulating cycles

~ improve pregnancy rates in women undergoing IVF.

In 2002 a team of German researchers discovered that acupuncture significantly increased the odds of pregnancy among a group of 160 women who were undergoing IVF treatment. Forty-two per cent of the women who received acupuncture got pregnant, compared to 26 per cent who did not. The researchers speculated that acupuncture helped to increase blood flow to the womb and relax the muscle tissue, giving the embryos a better chance of implanting. In 2006 researchers confirmed that acupuncture can significantly improve reproductive outcome in IVF.[62]

Other research suggests that acupuncture is effective in reducing stress which has been shown to interfere with hormonal balance. It makes sense that reducing your stress through acupuncture could theoretically improve your odds of conceiving. Some women find acupuncture helpful to cope with the stress they feel about trying to conceive.

Acupuncture may also help male infertility. New research shows that acupuncture can significantly improve the quality and health of sperm. In a study published in *Fertility and Sterility* in 2005, researchers analysed samples from men with infertility of unknown cause before and after acupuncture treatments. They found that acupuncture was associated with fewer structural defects in sperm and an increase in the number of normal sperm.[63]

HOMEOPATHY

Homeopathic remedies are designed to treat symptoms rather than conditions, as each case of a particular illness can manifest itself differently in different people. Before any drugs are prescribed to an individual, his or her medical history, family history, moods, likes, dislikes, sexual history and emotional state are all discussed thoroughly.

It is believed that in a person showing infertility signs the problems may not be directly related to the reproductive organs but to something less obvious, like an emotional condition, depression, fear of conceiving or dietary problems. Homeopathy eases these problems using plant, mineral or even metal sources. The pills prescribed are usually sweet and are taken at regular intervals throughout the day. Pulsatilla is often given for women with irregular or no periods and general remedies for infertility include lycopodium, argentums nitricum and selenenium metallicum. However, the remedies work best if – as with any complementary treatment – they are prescribed specifically and individually for the person concerned.

Several clinical trials have looked at the effects homeopathy can have on fertility.[64] Preliminary research has indicated that homeopathic treatment may not only help infertile women to achieve pregnancy but can also help to balance hormones and prevent miscarriage. Another study shows that homeopathy has potential for boosting fertility in men.[65]

Homeopathy is said to be one of the safest medical treatments with no known side effects, and may be a good option to treat infertility.

REFLEXOLOGY

Reflexology is based on the principle that there are certain reflex points on the feet, which are linked to different organs of the body via energy channels called meridians (as in Chinese medicine and acupuncture). When particular points are stimulated, they in turn stimulate specific body parts. The main use of reflexology is usually as a stress inhibitor, as it helps the whole body to relax and increase endorphin secretion, which elevates the feelgood factor.

The therapy itself feels like a vigorous foot massage. By pressuring one reflex point in the foot, the reflexologist influences the energy flow around the organs and body areas that run along that meridian.

Reflexology is particularly successful when used in conjunction with a healthy diet and lifestyle. Apart from relaxation, it can also boost blood circulation, help balance hormonal levels and regulate the menstrual cycle. It has also been found to be of assistance to those women suffering from endometriosis or PCOS.[66]

There has been little research done on the efficacy of reflexology in infertility, although a small trial in Denmark examined 108 women with an average age of 30 who had been trying to conceive for an average of 6.7 years. Many dropped out of the trial, but 19 of the remaining 61 conceived within six months of completing the treatment.[67]

HYPNOTHERAPY

Because the link between mind and body can be so strong, hypnotherapy works best for problems when there is a psychological component. Hypnotherapy works on the premise that there are two states of consciousness – the conscious and the subconscious – which may be at odds with each other. For example, a woman may say that she wants a baby but her subconscious fears may be preventing her from getting pregnant.

There is huge pressure on women these days to have the perfect body, job, partner and family. Many may have unacknowledged doubts and insecurities about motherhood and feel pressurised to conceive by those around them. It is important to find out what you really want because studies show that stress or anxiety about becoming a mother can prevent conception. Hypnotherapy can highlight and deal with any doubts you might have about your future role as a mother.[68]

The research on hypnotherapy and fertility is fragmented and often appears in medical journals in the form of single case studies of individual patients. Yet there is enough evidence to suggest that hypnotherapy can have an effect on fertility. This may be because, like visualisation, autogenic training (a form of thought control) and relaxation techniques, it works by harnessing the power of your mind to work for you, rather than against you.[69]

AROMATHERAPY

Aromatherapy is a natural treatment that uses the therapeutic properties of essential oils, extracted from the flowers, leaves, stems, bark or wood of aromatic plants and trees. Essential oils can be extremely potent concentrates that can be absorbed into the skin, hair and lungs, through massage, bathing and inhaling. Oils in the bloodstream will circulate for several hours, while those inhaled will stimulate the limbic system in the brain which deals with emotions.

Aromatherapists believe that certain oils can help to regulate hormonal imbalances and release stress which can also be contributory factors in infertility. Oils of particular relevance are: lavender, clary sage, geranium, jasmine, melissa, rose, sandalwood, neroli and ylang ylang which appear to affect the central nervous system and have a calming, antidepressant effect. Although there are no published studies of the benefits of aromatherapy for infertility there is research into aromatherapy for anxiety and other stress-related disorders.[70]

Note: because some oils (for example, fennel and anise) are not considered safe if you are pregnant (or hoping to be) always consult a qualified practitioner before self-medicating.

OSTEOPATHY

Osteopathy is a manual treatment that re-aligns the body through the musculoskeletal system to help the body's own self-healing mechanism.

Techniques are used to release underlying stresses and tension throughout the body. Some techniques can be very subtle and use light pressure as in cranial osteopathy while others use direct manipulation. Many osteopaths will use a combination of both, depending on the individual problem.

YOGA

Certain yoga positions have been known for ages to boost circulation to the reproductive system in both men and women. Because of the helpful properties of these positions, numerous yoga studios and mind/body classes have begun to incorporate fertility yoga into their routines.

THE BOTTOM LINE

Don't feel pressured in any way to try all or indeed any of these treatments. Remember that diet and lifestyle changes and supplement recommendations should be your prime focus and whether or not you decide to explore complementary therapies is totally up to you. From my perspective there are many good reasons to use complementary therapies to enhance your fertility, not least because they can be effective in apparently hopeless cases. However, they should not be used as a last-ditch alternative to orthodox medicine but as a complement to it. In my experience the best results are achieved when the two branches of medicine are working together for you.

MY TOP TEN GOLDEN FERTILITY-BOOSTING LIFESTYLE RULES

1   Encourage your partner to eat healthily and make positive lifestyle changes with you.
2   If you or your partner smoke – quit.
3   If either of you drinks – stop.
4   Find ways to fit exercise into your life.
5   Make quality sleep a priority.
6   Have lots of sex – and make sure you enjoy it.
7   Find ways to manage stress and be good to yourself.
8   Don't put your life on hold.
9   Support your partner and let your partner, friends and loved ones support you; get help from a professional if needed.
10 Use complementary therapies to add to the benefits of what you are doing with the nutritional side.

step three
fertility-*boosting*
supplements

A healthy diet is the ideal basis for good health, but because nowadays it is not so easy to get all the fertility-boosting nutrients you need from your diet, taking supplements may be extremely beneficial.

With the dominance of supermarket shopping, there's no way of knowing the freshness or nutritional content of the food you buy. Even if you choose all the right foods it is likely that much of their nutritional value will have been stripped by modern agricultural and production processes.[1] For example, almost 80 per cent of zinc is removed from wheat during the milling process to ensure that bread has longer shelf life.[2]

Part of the problem is that the soil food is grown on today is so lacking in nutrients due to overuse and commercial farming methods, so that even foods we regard as healthy, like vegetables, may not contain the nutrients you expect. According to joint research by the Royal Society of Chemistry and the Ministry of Agriculture, Fisheries and Food, between 1940 and 1990 vegetables lost 76 per cent of their copper content, 24 per cent of their magnesium and 27 per cent of their iron. From the vitamin point of view, in the time between an orange being picked and the time you eat it, most of its vitamin C will be lost.

It's clear that many of us are simply not getting all the nutrients we need to ensure optimum health and fertility from our food. This was confirmed by a National Diet and Nutritional survey published in 2003 that looked at adults aged 19–64 and showed that only 15 per cent of women and 13 per cent of men actually met the five-a-day target for fruit and vegetables. Seventy-four per cent of women failed to achieve the Reference Nutrient Intake (RNI) for magnesium, 45 per cent for zinc, 84 per cent for folic acid and 15 per cent for vitamin D.

Add to these statistics the effects of additives, preservatives and toxins (see Steps 1 and 4) in your food and you can see how it can have a damaging effect on your fertility. You've seen how important it is to take in the right amount of nutrients in the pre-conception period, so to ensure that you really do get all that you need I strongly advise taking supplements.

All the supplements outlined in this chapter have been shown to be highly effective for optimum nutrition, fertility boosting and a healthy pregnancy in conjunction with (not instead of) a healthy diet.

FOLIC ACID

An essential B vitamin, folic acid (folate) is absolutely crucial for a healthy pregnancy, but it is also one of the vitamins in which we are most commonly deficient. Your body needs folic acid to produce DNA. Folic acid protects the neural tube – which will go on to form the spine and spinal cord – and helps to close it properly to ensure normal brain and spinal cord function. Folic acid can help to protect an unborn baby from developing spina bifida (an abnormal development of the spinal cord) and anencephaly (absence of most of the brain). The neural tube should close between the 25th and 30th day after conception, when women may still not realise they are pregnant which is why all women trying to get pregnant should take folic acid each day and up to three months before conception.[3]

Doctors will always recommend folic acid when a woman says she is trying for a baby. What a lot of doctors and women don't know, however, is that supplementing with folic acid alone is not enough. This is because folic acid and vitamins B6 and B12 are interlinked and to work effectively you must have enough of each of them.

The very latest research into heart disease suggests that folic acid and vitamins B6 and B12 may also help to control an amino acid called homocysteine that damages the lining of blood cells. Since high levels of homocysteine are also found in women who have miscarriages, supplementing with these vitamins makes sense.[4]

When trying to get pregnant, be aware that folic acid deficiency is likely in people with chronic diarrhoea or digestive disorders. Alcohol also causes the body to lose folic acid as do certain drugs and oral contraceptives. Vegetarians and vegans are also more likely to have deficiencies in vitamin B12 than people who eat animal produce.

Your partner should also consider taking folic acid supplements as new evidence suggests that folic acid deficiency reduces fertility in men and may damage the DNA carried by sperm. After showing that a folate-restricted diet made sperm counts plunge by 90 per cent in rats, researcher Bruce Ames and his colleagues at the University of California at Berkeley showed that folic acid deficiency has a similar effect in men.[5]
Dose: both you and your partner should take 400µg a day of folic acid, along with vitamin B6 (20mg) and vitamin B12 (20µg).

ZINC

Zinc deficiency is another problem that I often come across when testing in the clinic. It is crucial for your fertility and is the most widely studied fertility-boosting nutrient for both men and women. It is an essential component of genetic material and a deficiency can lead to reduced fertility, hormone imbalance and an increased risk of miscarriage.[6]

Zinc is vitally important for growth and proper cell division in a foetus. During IVF treatment, after the egg has fertilised the doctors have to wait for the cells to divide before putting it back into a woman; the same cell division takes place in a natural pregnancy. Without optimum zinc levels, not only is it difficult to conceive but there are risks that the baby may be born with malformations or poor brain and nervous system development.[7]

Zinc is also needed for the proper development of sperm. Research suggests that zinc deficiency in men causes a temporary but reversible reduction in sperm count and a reduced testosterone level; giving zinc to men with low testosterone levels increases sperm count.[8] Other studies comparing men with low sperm counts with those whose sperm counts are normal show that zinc levels are significantly lower in men with low sperm counts. What's more, with each ejaculation men lose up to 9 per cent of their daily zinc intake, so it is important that men keep up a good daily intake of zinc.[9]

Other symptoms of zinc deficiency include white spots on the nails, irregular periods and a poor sense of taste and smell.

Dose: for fertility boosting you and your partner are advised to take 30mg zinc a day. Make sure it is in the form of zinc acsorbate or zinc citrate as these are more easily absorbed than the inorganic forms e.g. sulphate or oxide.

SELENIUM

This mineral is used to make antioxidants called selenoproteins which help protect your body from free radical damage – very important in the process of cell division. With its protective effect selenium can prevent chromosome breakage which is known to cause birth defects and miscarriages. Deficiency in women has been linked to a higher risk of miscarriage.[10]

Good levels of selenium are also essential for sperm formation and testosterone production in men.[11] A lack of selenium in men is associated with sperm that cannot move properly, selenium being essential for making their strong whiplash tails. In one double-blind trial selenium supplementation resulted in an increase in fertility from 17.5 to 35.1 per cent in sub-fertile men. Other studies show that blood selenium levels are lower in men with low sperm counts.[12]

Research suggests that the antioxidant activity of selenium may even make sperm more fertile. An interesting study looked at men with good sperm counts but low fertilisation rates during IVF treatments. They were given selenium and vitamin E supplements each day and one month after starting treatment their fertility rate increased from 19 per cent to 29 per cent.[13]

Selenium is a mineral that should be in our soil where we grow our food but due to modern farming methods this is not always the case. As selenium deficiency shows no obvious signs, it is safer and wiser to supplement.

Dose: both you and your partner should take 100µg of selenium a day.

ESSENTIAL FATTY ACIDS (EFAs)

Over the last century there has been an 80 per cent decrease in the consumption of omega 3 fatty acids;[14] it is now thought that we are getting too many omega 6 fats from our diet and not enough omega 3s.

Omega 3 fats are important for regulating reproductive hormones and boosting your baby's brain, eye and central nervous system development.

From essential fatty acids you produce beneficial prostaglandins which have hormone-like functions. They are believed to prevent low birth weight and decrease the likelihood of premature birth.[15] Fish oil has also been shown to help prevent blood from clotting inappropriately so it can be beneficial to women in whom recurrent miscarriages have been linked to a clotting problem (see page 173).[16]

For men, essential fatty acid supplementation is important because semen is rich in the prostaglandins produced from these fats. Research has shown that men who have problems with abnormal sperm tend to have lower than normal levels of beneficial prostaglandins.[17]

Because our Western diet is usually high in omega 6s, found in abundance in many vegetables oils, you should decrease your intake of vegetable oils and boost your intake of less abundant omega 3s.

The Department of Health recommends that we should all double our intake of omega 3s by eating oily fish (such as salmon) two to three times a week and more green, leafy vegetables and beans. But more and more research indicates that it is wise to supplement with these fatty acids and not to rely on dietary intake. That's why I encourage all couples trying for a baby to start supplementing with essential fatty acids several months before conception.

To avoid ingesting harmful toxins and chemicals from the bones, skin and connective tissue of animals that may have been pumped full of chemicals, make sure the capsules the fish oil is contained in are made of fish gelatine and not bovine (cattle) gelatine. But whatever fish oil you choose, avoid cod liver oil capsules. Fish often absorb toxins and chemicals and oil taken from the liver – the organ of detoxification – is likely to have higher quantities. Several companies have had to take theirs off the shelves as they contained very high levels of toxins called dioxins. Cod liver oil also contains high levels of vitamin A which, in this form, is not recommended during pregnancy.

If you are a vegetarian or prefer not to take fish oil the best way to supplement omega 3 fatty acids is by taking flax (linseed) oil capsules. Linseed oil contains both omega 3 and 6 EFAs. The body has to convert linseed oil to EPA (eicosapentaenoic acid) and DHA (docosahexaenoic acid), both of which are needed for fertility. DHA is also important for your baby's health. It is estimated that from linseed (flax) oil only 5–10 per cent is converted to EPA and 2–5 per cent for DHA, so if you are not vegetarian, fish oil is preferable.

Symptoms of EFA deficiency include dry skin, dry hair, depression, poor concentration, weight gain and menstrual irregularity.

Dose: both you and your partner should take a supplement containing at least 600–700mg of EPA a day. The omega 3 supplement should also contain good amounts of DHA (at least 500mg a day), essential for the baby's eye and central nervous system development once you get pregnant. (I recommend Omega 3 Plus.)

Note: don't be misled by labels on supplements that say 'fish oil 1000mg' or 'omega 3 1000mg' – you need to read the breakdown of EPA and DHA to know what you are getting. Try also to ensure the fish oil you buy is in its 'natural triglyceride' form as in the original fish. Or take linseed (flax) oil 1000mg. You can get vegetarian sources of EPA and DHA from algae but the levels of EPA and DHA are quite low.

VITAMIN B6

Vitamin B6 is important for the development and maintenance of a healthy immune system and consequently protects against cancer as well as infection. It can help to prevent damage to chromosomes which is obviously crucial at the point of conception. Many women use vitamin B6 for the relief of premenstrual syndrome and irregular periods with some success and it also plays a critical role in fertility. In addition, vitamin B6 is intricately involved in the function of many enzymes and in protein metabolism and formation.[18]

Research has shown that giving vitamin B6 to women who have trouble conceiving can help to regularise periods and increase fertility. In one study 12 out of 14 women who had been trying to conceive did so after taking vitamin B6 daily for six months.[19]

Vitamin B6 deficiency may result in poor immune function, hormone imbalances and various other problems. Lack of vitamin B6 also reduces vitamin B12 absorption and utilisation and may contribute to B12 deficiency. Signs of vitamin B6 deficiency

include skin problems (especially dry skin), rashes and oily, scaly skin around scalp, eyebrows and behind ears, PMS, morning sickness, fluid retention and insomnia.
Dose: both you and your partner should take up to 20mg of vitamin B6 a day.

VITAMIN B12

Vitamin B12 is probably the best known of all the vitamins, with recognised deficiency symptoms, most obviously pernicious anaemia. It is water-soluble so the body is unable to store extensive amounts of this vitamin and must therefore get a regular supply from the diet. This can be difficult for some people, either because they absorb vitamin B12 poorly or because their diet is deficient, especially in the case of vegans.

Vitamin B12 is vital for cellular reproduction and a number of studies have shown its potential for reducing the risk of miscarriage[20] and raising low sperm count.
Dose: both you and your partner should take up to 20µg of vitamin B12 a day.

VITAMIN E

Discovered in 1922 through experiments with rats, this powerful antioxidant contains tocopherols, a Greek word meaning to bear children. Scientists discovered that rats without vitamin E in their diet became infertile. In a preliminary human trial, infertile couples given vitamin E showed a significant increase in fertility.[21]

Vitamin E's beneficial role in female reproductive health has since been backed up by more recent research and it has even been suggested that it may reduce age-related ovarian decline.[22]

For men, vitamin E – like other antioxidants – combats free radicals, high levels of which can lower sperm count. So it is important to ensure adequate intake of antioxidants, especially vitamin E. Research[23] suggests that the antioxidant activity of vitamin E may make sperm more fertile.

If you have been diagnosed with unexplained infertility I recommend that you and your partner take vitamin E supplements and also if you have had a miscarriage because it can prevent abnormal clotting. Studies have shown that giving vitamin E to both partners can result in significant increases in fertility.[24]

Symptoms of vitamin E deficiency include irritability and anaemia.
Dose: both you and your partner should take up to 160mg natural rather than synthetic vitamin E a day. Normally natural and synthetic vitamins are of equal value but with vitamin E the two forms are structurally different. A study in the *American Journal of Clinical Nutrition* looked at the effects of both natural (d-alpha-tocopherol) and synthetic (dl-alpha- tocopherol) vitamin E and found that the absorption rate of the natural version was more efficient than the synthetic.[25]

VITAMIN C

This key antioxidant keeps your body, including your reproductive organs, running efficiently. Although animals manufacture vitamin C in their bodies we don't, which means we have to get it from our diet.

Research in the 1970s showed that when vitamin C was given to women undergoing fertility treatment it helped to trigger ovulation and recent research confirms its crucial role.[26] It appears that if vitamin C is taken at the same time as fertility drugs, such as clomiphene, it can help to trigger ovulation, even in women who might not respond to the drug.

Studies have also established that deficiencies in vitamin C can decrease sperm quality. In one study, when a group of men had their vitamin C intake reduced from 250mg a day to 5mg a day their sperm had double the normal DNA damage. In another it was shown that supplementing with 1000mg of vitamin C increased sperm quality and quantity. Vitamin C reduces agglutination (when sperm stick together, affecting fertility), and in a controlled study, supplementation with 100–200mg of vitamin C a day increased fertility in men with this condition.[27] Men with normal sperm results, i.e. a good count, motility and normal sperm, have much higher levels of vitamin C when measured in semen compared to men who have problem sperm.[28] It appears that vitamin C has a protective effect on sperm DNA and it is thought that DNA damage can make it difficult to conceive and increase the risk of miscarriage.[29]

Symptoms of vitamin C deficiency include fatigue and lowered immunity.

Dose: both you and your partner should take 500mg of vitamin C twice a day. Vitamin C is better split into two doses as it is water-soluble and excreted every few hours. When buying vitamin C supplements, choose the ascorbate form (such as magnesium or calcium ascorbate); this is a buffered (non-acidic) form and is gentler on the stomach than ascorbic acid, the most common form of vitamin C. Also you are aiming for your body and cervical mucus to be more alkaline (see page 131) so it is better to avoid the more acidic form.

MANGANESE

Manganese, a trace mineral that plays a part in many enzyme systems in the body, is needed for healthy skin, bone and cartilage formation and to regulate blood sugar levels. It was first considered an essential nutrient in 1931. Researchers discovered that experimental animals fed a diet deficient in manganese demonstrated poor growth and impaired reproduction.

Manganese is essential for the proper functioning of an enzyme called superoxide dismutase (SOD), crucial for controlling free radical damage which causes us to age more quickly and creates inflammation in the body. So manganese is an important mineral for fertility, when we are aiming to improve the quality of both eggs and sperm and to control abnormal DNA changes which might stop a pregnancy continuing.

Manganese deficiency is associated with nausea, vomiting, poor glucose tolerance (high blood sugar levels), skin rash, loss of hair colour, excessive bone loss, low cholesterol levels, dizziness, hearing loss and compromised function of the reproductive system.

Dose: both you and your partner should take 5mg of manganese a day.

IRON

Iron is vital to the health of the human body and is found in every human cell, primarily linked with protein to form the oxygen-carrying molecule haemoglobin. Without iron new cells would not be produced and your body would not get the oxygen it needs to survive. That's why iron deficiency causes tiredness because your body is being starved of oxygen.

Taking iron is known to help women regain their fertility[30] and iron supplements taken together with vitamin C (which increases the absorption of iron) can further boost fertility.[31]

Symptoms of iron deficiency include a sore tongue, fatigue, hair loss, pale complexion, heavy periods and breathlessness.

Note: supplementation with iron is not necessary if you have not been diagnosed with a deficiency and your doctor can test you for this. Haem iron – the most absorbable form – is found in animal produce, such as fish and poultry. Non-haem iron is found in leafy green vegetables and dried fruit. Apart from eating these iron-rich foods you can increase your intake of iron naturally by not drinking tea with food (the tannin contained in tea can block the uptake of iron and other important nutrients). Iron intake can also be increased by cooking foods in iron or stainless steel pans; aluminium should be avoided as it can deplete the iron content of food.

L-ARGININE

Amino acids have been proven to be important supplements for men in addressing infertility problems. The head of the sperm contains a large amount of L-arginine – an amino acid found in many foods and one that is essential for sperm production. A great deal of research has shown that L-arginine deficiency should be considered when there are problems with sperm and male fertility. Studies suggest that increasing levels of L-arginine can increase sperm count and quality.[32]

Supplementation with L-arginine has also been shown to improve fertilisation rates in women with a previous history of failed attempts at IVF[33] but the research is only preliminary and until we know more only your partner should supplement with it. **Dose:** your partner only should take around 300mg of L-arginine a day.

L-CARNITINE

Another amino acid that appears to be crucial for healthy sperm function is L-carnitine and studies have shown that supplementing with it helped to increase sperm count.[34] **Dose:** your partner only should take 100mg of L-carnitine a day.

CO-ENZYME Q10

This is a vitamin-like substance that is contained in nearly every cell of the body. It is important for energy production and normal carbohydrate metabolism (the way the body breaks down the carbohydrates you eat in order to turn it into energy). Because of its role in energy production it is a significant nutrient for men if sperm motility is poor. Co-enzyme Q10 is concentrated in the area between the head and tail of the sperm; the energy for movement and all other energy-dependent processes in the sperm cell depend on it. Lower levels of co-enzyme Q10 have been found in men with poor sperm motility[35] and supplementing with this nutrient led to a significant improvement.[36]

As co-enzyme Q10 also functions as an antioxidant it can be helpful for sperm cells to protect membranes from free radical damage so would be suggested for those who have a higher proportion of abnormal sperm or high DNA sperm damage. **Dose:** your partner can take up to 60mg of co-enzyme Q10 a day.

VITAMIN A

This is an essential antioxidant, which not only protects the mucus membranes – including those in the reproductive tract – from infection, but also safeguards against cell mutations. High doses of retinol (the animal form of vitamin A, found in liver) can increase the risk of having a handicapped baby but the vegetable sources of vitamin A (beta carotene) found in carrots, tomatoes, cabbage and broccoli do not cause defects and are therefore a much safer way to get your vitamin A.[37] **Dose:** if you're trying to get pregnant, beta carotene is safe to take as a supplement. You can take up to 15mg of beta-carotene a day, although 5mg is enough.

TESTING FOR MINERAL DEFICIENCIES A simple hair test can be carried out to check if you have any mineral deficiencies (see page 218). A while back a farmer and his wife came to see me. They had visited an IVF clinic that morning who said that they didn't test for minerals. The farmer told me that he breeds prize cattle and takes blood samples from the herd to be tested at a lab for deficiencies. The lab tell him how much zinc and selenium to add to the feed to increase the fertility of the cattle and produce the healthiest offspring. The farmer commented that he could not understand why we do not routinely do this for humans!

MY STORY After a hair mineral test for both of us, you devised an eating plan and vitamins and minerals that we needed. Since then we had ICSI treatment and had a little girl. After her birth, I followed your programme again because I wanted another baby. This time we conceived naturally. So thank you very much for all your help. We would not be a family without it. I am positive that with your help ICSI worked for us the first time, so thank you for that too.

TRY HERBAL HELPERS

In addition to vitamin and mineral supplements you may also find it helpful to try fertility-boosting herbal remedies.

Herbs are the oldest form of medicine and are the foundation for many pharmaceutical drugs. For example, aspirin was originally extracted from willow bark. The following herbs can be helpful for boosting fertility but should only be used under the guidance of a qualified practitioner, as in my clinics where they are tailored to the individual needs of the couple. I use specific herbs for certain conditions such as PCOS, endometriosis, fibroids and so on, but the herbs mentioned below are more general.

Note: if you are taking drugs as part of your fertility treatment, you should not take any herbs but continue with nutritional supplements. Any herb should be used with caution during pregnancy.

AGNUS CASTUS

Agnus castus (vitex/chasteberry tree) has been shown[38] to stimulate and normalise the function of the pituitary gland which in turn helps to balance hormone output from the ovaries and stimulate ovulation.

Agnus castus also keeps prolactin secretion in check (excessive prolactin can prevent ovulation). It is useful as a herbal treatment for infertility, particularly in cases with established luteal phase defect (shortened second half of the menstrual cycle) and high levels of the hormone prolactin. In one trial, 48 women (aged between 23 and 39) diagnosed with infertility took agnus castus once daily for three months. Seven became pregnant during the trial and 25 experienced normalised progesterone levels – which may increase the chances for pregnancy.[39]

Agnus castus works to restore hormone balance (it is classed as an adaptogen which means it has a balancing effect) and can help encourage ovulation, regulate periods, restart periods that have stopped, ease heavy bleeding and painful periods and increase the ratio of progesterone to oestrogen by balancing excess oestrogen. If you have been told that you have a hormone imbalance or that your periods are irregular it is well worth taking it over a few months.

DONG QUAI (ANGELICA SINENSIS)

This oriental herb, also called Angelica Sinensis, is well known as a tonic for the female reproductive system that can help to regulate hormones and encourage the normal function of the sex organs.[40]

DAMIANA (TURNERA DIFFUSA)

This herb is a good male tonic and can be helpful where there is reduced sex drive, impotence or problems with ejaculation.

GINKGO BILOBA

Known for its beneficial effects on circulation and blood flow, this herb can be helpful where there are problems getting and keeping an erection.[41] It is thought that ginkgo improves sexual performance by releasing nitric oxide in the penis which helps with an erection. Ginkgo is also thought to help with sex drive.

SIBERIAN GINSENG (ELEUTHEROCOCCUS SENTICOSUS)

Siberian ginseng is an excellent herb for people under a lot of stress. It has a long history in helping with adrenal function and calming the body. Siberian ginseng is classed as an adaptogen – it provides energy when required and helps to combat stress and fatigue when somebody is under pressure. It helps to encourage the normal functioning of the adrenals and acts as a tonic to these glands.[42]

TAKING YOUR SUPPLEMENTS

At this stage you may well be wondering how on earth you and your partner are going to be able to take all these supplements! But it's not as difficult as you may think if you can find a multivitamin and mineral designed specifically for fertility and pregnancy.

There is a tendency for certain vitamins and minerals to be hyped in the press but one nutrient is not more important than the other. Individual supplements can be effective in rebalancing your hormones and improving health and fertility, but since all nutrients depend on each other to function properly, you should take a high-quality multivitamin and mineral on a daily basis as the basic foundation and then, if needed, take other nutrients on top.

According to research from the University of Leeds women who take daily multivitamin tablets can double their chances of getting pregnant as, they believe, it can help to produce better-quality eggs. A study presented to the European Society of Human Reproduction in July 2001 showed that in 215 women undergoing IVF in Leeds *and* taking the multivitamin pill, the fluid surrounding the eggs was enriched with vitamins C and E which, the researchers believe, can give the egg a crucial boost. Leader of the research, gynaecology senior registrar Dr Sara Matthews, said: 'My theory is that it might apply to anyone trying for pregnancy.'[43]

SUMMARY OF REQUIRED DOSES IN SUPPLEMENTS
FOR BOTH YOU AND HIM

~ Folic acid: 400µg
~ Zinc: 30mg
~ Selenium: 100µg
~ Vitamin B6: 20mg
~ Vitamin B3: 20mg
~ Vitamin B5: 20mg
~ Vitamin B1: 20mg
~ Vitamin B12: 20µg
~ Vitamin E: 160mg
~ Vitamin C: 1000 mg
~ Vitamin D: 2.5µg
~ Beta carotene: up to 5mg
~ Manganese: 5 mg
~ Chromium: 20µg
~ L-arginine: he needs 300 mg
~ L-carnitine: he needs 100 mg
~ **Either** fish oil: 600–700mg EPA and 500mg DHA
~ **Or** linseed oil (if you can't take fish): 1000mg

A good multivitamin and mineral supplement designed specifically for fertility will include 400µg of folic acid so you don't need to add in extra folic acid. (I use Fertility Plus for Women in the clinic as it contains everything mentioned above and in the right amounts). Your partner should also take a good multivitamin and mineral supplement for men, like Fertility Plus for Men. This also contains the extra arginine and carnitine. You would both then take vitamin C (as ascorbate, the alkaline form – the one I use in the clinic is Vitamin C Plus) and a good fish oil capsule (containing good levels of both EPA and DHA, such as Omega 3 Plus).

If you have difficulty getting Fertility Plus, Omega 3 Plus or Vitamin C Plus locally, then go to *www.naturalhealthpractice.com* or phone the contact number on page 218). *Note:* it's important to remember that a huge range of nutrients is important for your fertility and many have yet to be discovered. Although in these days of refined foods you need to take supplements to make up for any shortfalls in your diet, they will never be a substitute for a varied and healthy diet. In a nutshell, you can't eat junk food and take supplements and expect to be in the best of health. Supplements are, as their name suggests, 'supplementary' to your diet and are designed to give you a boost while you are eating well, for the best possible chance of getting pregnant quickly.

AN ADDED BONUS By now you should have started to make changes in your diet and lifestyle to boost your fertility and hopefully taking quality supplements will be one of these changes. What you may not appreciate at this early stage is that all the recommendations in Steps 1 to 3 won't only boost your fertility – they will boost your general health and well-being too. In just a few weeks you will notice that you feel more relaxed and upbeat, you'll have better digestion, fewer aches and pains, softer skin, brighter eyes and bags of energy. All this is an unexpected but commonly reported bonus of following my fertility-boosting three-month plan.

step four
eliminate
environmental and occupational hazards

Where you work and what you are exposed to on a daily basis can have an impact on how quickly you become pregnant. Like stress, it is very difficult to quantify exactly the impact of environmental factors on fertility, but if you want to get pregnant faster you need to be armed with as much information as possible.

This chapter discusses the suggested links between occupational and environmental hazards and infertility with advice on what you can do to protect against them. Some are easier to address than others, but you can decide what's realistic for you and make beneficial changes or modifications accordingly.

EVERYDAY TOXINS

Every day a cloud of potentially hormone-disturbing toxins surrounds us: pesticides and herbicides in our soil, chemicals and additives in the food we eat, contaminants in the water we drink, pollutants from car exhausts and cigarette smoke, chemicals in solvents, plastics and adhesives, as well as all those we absorb through our skin in make-up, hair dyes and household cleaning products (along with possible radiation from mobile phones or VDUs).

According to a recent Friends of the Earth press briefing for safer chemicals campaign there are now over 300 chemicals which didn't exist 50 years ago that can collect in our bodies, rob us of fertility-boosting nutrients and interfere with hormonal health.[1]

We are getting a strong hint about the detrimental effects of toxins and pollutants on our health and fertility from the animal world. Infertility in wildlife is thought to be linked to substances known as xenoestrogens – oestrogen-like substances in the environment caused by pollution from pesticides and the manufacturing of plastics.

Research in 2002 from Brunel University reported on a five-year study which found sex changes in male fish in UK rivers contaminated with synthetic (man-made) oestrogens or EDCs (endocrine-disrupting chemicals). Scientists blame the pollution on a 'potent' form of oestrogen found in urine from women using the contraceptive pill and HRT, which may be flushed through sewage works and into rivers. One could argue that this is evidence enough that we are living in a sea of oestrogen, a chemical cocktail, and that there are legitimate reasons to be worried about health and fertility.

Other studies show that pesticides, plastics and everyday substances such as additives, preservatives, cigarettes, fatty foods, alcohol and coffee contain toxins that upset our hormones and increase the risk of infertility and even cancer. And women exposed to heavy metals such as lead, aluminium and cadmium are more likely to have irregular periods and experience hormone imbalances and miscarriages or take longer to get pregnant.[2]

The harsh truth is that environmental and occupational toxins are threatening our health and damaging our fertility with a new kind of pollution.[3] Our bodies have to work extremely hard to process (metabolise) and get rid of (detoxify) them through the liver, kidneys, lymph and digestive system and, in doing so, we lose vital fertility-boosting nutrients.

The cause of many infertility cases (up to 30 per cent) remains 'unexplained' and it is my belief that, along with stress and poor nutrition, low-level exposure to everyday toxins may eventually be found to be the culprit.

ENDOCRINE-DISRUPTING CHEMICALS (EDCS) AND XENOESTROGENS

Everyday toxins have been linked to birth defects and hormonal disruption so great that some are called endocrine-disrupting chemicals. It is thought that EDCs could be interfering with your ability to conceive due to the damage they cause to your menstrual cycle and possibly your eggs, as well as to a man's sperm production. Experts aren't entirely sure how they threaten fertility but it appears that they have the potential to interfere with hormone production, preventing the required responses in much the same way that a car parked across an exit prevents other cars from getting in and out. They create havoc by tricking your body into a state of hormonal imbalance known as oestrogen excess or oestrogen dominance.

EDCs mimic our own natural hormones. They are stored in body fat and are found in everything from plastics to pesticides and the residues of hormonal medications that don't break down once they pass into our water supply. Although the government tells us EDCs are safe, there is a strong body of evidence to suggest that they are not and that they have potentially damaging effects on hormonal health and health in general.[4]

It's no coincidence, in my opinion, that there has been a huge proliferation of xenoestrogens in the last 20 years and a decrease in sperm counts of 50 per cent, an increase in testicular cancer, earlier onset of puberty in girls and an increased number of boys born with undescended testes and other problems with their reproductive organs.

YOUR VERY OWN CHEMICAL CLEARING HOUSE

A toxin is any substance that is detrimental to cell functioning and the overall health of your body and, as we've seen, there are thousands of new ones in the environment. These are putting a huge and daily burden on your detoxifying organs (your liver and kidneys). Although you can limit your exposure, it's virtually impossible to avoid toxins altogether in today's busy, industrialised world. So you and your partner need to fortify yourselves against the effects of unavoidable exposure by keeping your detoxifying organs in good working order so that toxins are successfully expelled from your system.

Your liver is your very own chemical clearing house. Every minute of the day it cleans one and a half quarts of blood so that other organs can be nourished with purified blood. It also neutralises toxic wastes, sending them off to your kidneys for elimination and removes excess hormones such as oestrogen, thereby maintaining hormonal balance. In addition, it produces amino acids and enzymes to metabolise fat, proteins and carbohydrates and helps to regulate blood sugar levels for energy.

If toxins clog up your liver's detoxification pathways, your blood sugar levels start to fluctuate, toxins find their way into your circulatory system, excess hormones can't be cleared from your system and symptoms of hormone imbalance are likely to occur. And when your liver is overloaded it will also force your kidneys and adrenals to work overtime. But the more pressure there is on your adrenal glands to cope with unwanted toxins, the greater the likelihood that there will be overproduction of cortisol (see page 63) – another trigger for reproductive hormone imbalances.

To keep your in-house detoxification system in good working order you need to find ways to cleanse both your diet and your lifestyle.

CLEANSE YOUR DIET

A nutrient-rich, preferably organic, diet that excludes alcohol, smoking and caffeine – all of which can have a toxic effect on your body – is the best way to protect yourself and your fertility from toxic damage.[5]

It is especially important to ensure you are getting enough antioxidant-rich foods in your diet. Research has shown how powerful the detoxifying effects of antioxidants such as vitamins A, E and C and selenium can be. Another beneficial nutrient for your liver is sulphur – garlic, cruciferous vegetables and eggs are all good sources.

As you eat healthily, you will also lose weight if needed, but what I am suggesting is that you clean up your diet, *not* that you embark on a radical detox or that you lose weight too quickly. If you do either of these, toxins can be released quickly into the bloodstream and as you are aiming to boost your fertility over just three months you do not want to be flooding your body with toxins at this crucial time. Normal rates of fat loss will give a slow release and your body will cope with them fine.

So if you and your partner are eating a healthy, antioxidant-rich diet according to my fertility-boosting diet guidelines in Step 1 you will already be giving your body the most effective form of defence against unwanted environmental toxins.

CLEANSE YOUR LIFE

The next step is to reduce the amount of toxins you're exposed to on a daily basis and the guidelines below will help you to do just that.

Protect yourself from pesticides

When you pile your plate with vegetables you get a load of nutrients on the plus side, but you may also get the pesticides, insecticides and other chemicals used to protect crops from bugs, rodents and bacteria. And if you use pesticides in your garden or to protect your pets from fleas or to rid your house of insects or rodents you are exposed to even more. They can also be found in some plastics, household products and industrial chemicals. It's estimated that around 3,900 different brands of pesticides are used on food, on pets or in homes. Some fruit and vegetables are sprayed ten times before they reach the shops.[6]

Pesticides are potent, extremely toxic, chemicals that can interfere with hormonal health in both men and women.[7] One study looking at male partners at a Massachusetts infertility clinic suggests that a common pesticide sprayed on food and also used in insect killers can suppress levels of testosterone and possibly affect fertility. Spot urine samples showed that men with high levels of pesticide residues had reduced testosterone levels by up to 10 per cent.[8]

The following simple strategies will help you to protect yourself from unnecessary exposure to pesticides:

~ Use home, lawn and garden pesticides sparingly or better still not at all; if you have to use them don't handle them in the three months prior to conception.

~ Don't have your house treated for woodworm in the three months prior to conception.

~ Treat pets for fleas with natural herbal sprays or ask your vet about other natural ways to deal with them. If you crush garlic tablets in your pet's food this can keep the fleas away.

~ Investigate natural insect repellents; again, garlic can work wonders.

~ Rinse but don't soak fresh fruit and vegetables; this is a more effective way to remove pesticide residue.

~ Wash and peel non-organic fruit and vegetables before using them. Remove and discard the outer leaves of cabbages and other greens. Safe vegetable washes are available at health food shops or you can simply use a few teaspoons of vinegar in a bowl of water. Washing can't alter any pesticides absorbed in the vegetables but peeling fruit and vegetables can lower residues by about three quarters. If you buy organic, however, you need only scrub the skins.

~ Eat a wide variety of fruit and vegetables as specific pesticides are used for specific crops and this way you'll avoid eating too much of a given pesticide.

~ Make sure you are getting enough fibre (see page 18) because it helps to prevent the absorption of toxins into the bloodstream.

~ Buy organic food whenever possible (see page 29). Find out where to buy pesticide-free organically grown food in your community – one taste and you'll go back for more. A great variety of organically grown food can also be ordered online.

~ If you must eat meat, only eat organic (see page 31). Organically produced meat is produced without the routine use of drugs common in intensive livestock farming.

~ It goes without saying that you should avoid any food that is genetically modified. The BSE beef crisis was lesson enough but research has also shown that GM foods affect the fertility of insects and that you cannot manipulate natural food without consequences to your health.

Protect yourself from plastics

We drink from plastic bottles and use plastic food wraps all the time but concern among scientists is growing about the safety of these products, as well as tin cans and dental sealants. This is because substances in certain plastics have been shown to have EDCs such as nonylphenol and octylphenol, biphenolic compounds and phthalates.

One such chemical is bisphenol A, a synthetic oestrogen used in the manufacture of many food containers, cans, baby bottles and dental sealants. An illustration of the power of this chemical is that some male workers developed breasts after inhaling dust containing bisphenol A and one study showed that women with a history of miscarriage can have as much as three times the chemical bisphenol A in their blood as women who have never miscarried.[9]

Studies have raised questions about the safety of cling film made of a type of plastic called polyvinyl chloride (PVC) containing plasticisers. Some research suggests that PVC may be an endocrine disruptor.[10] Other research on phthalates (used as softeners of plastics, solvents in perfumes and additives to hair sprays, lubricants and insect repellents) has shown that they have the potential to be reproductive toxins.[11]

Until more is known about the effects of common plastics on our health use the simple strategies below to protect yourself:

~ Use plastic wraps and cookware made of polyethylene which doesn't contain plasticisers. If the product doesn't make this clear, don't buy it.
~ When you reheat or cook food don't let plastic wrap touch it.
~ Don't wrap food in cling film; use paper instead. Immediately remove cling film wrap from any food you buy and transfer it to a bag or container.
~ Don't store fatty food in plastic wrap. Xenoestrogens are lipophilic (fat loving) and will tend to leach into foods with a high fat content.
~ If you buy hard cheese wrapped in plastic use a knife to shave off the surface layer.
~ Do not microwave food in plastic containers; better still avoid microwaving altogether.
~ Use glass bottles. Cans and plastic bottles of fizzy drink contain six times the amount of aluminium compared to the same beverages in glass bottles. There is always a small amount of residue that dissolves into drinks from the lining of a can or from a plastic bottle.
~ Refill your own non-plastic water bottle instead of using toxic plastic water bottles. While it's good for your health to carry your own water and drink it throughout the day, if it's in a clear polycarbonate plastic bottle, it is leaching a toxic substance into your water – even if the bottle is sitting on the table at room temperature.

Spot hidden ingredients
Getting used to spotting hidden ingredients is a good way to avoid toxins and chemicals. Additives in food have been linked to health problems such as headaches, asthma, allergies and hyperactivity in kids, hormone imbalances and even cancer.

The following should make understanding labels easier:

Colourings A dangerous class of additives and one of the easiest to avoid. Look at labels for: artificial colour added, the words green, blue or yellow followed by a number, colour added with no explanation, tartrazine (E102), Quinoline yellow (E104), Sunset yellow (E110), Beetroot red (E162), Caramel (E150) or FD and C red no 3.

Some foods contain natural colours obtained from plants and these are safe. The most common is annatto, from the reddish seed of a tropical tree. Annatto is often added to cheese to make it more orange or butter to make it more yellow. Red pigments obtained from beets, green from chlorella and carotene from carrots are also fine.

Preservatives The main function of preservatives is to extend a food's shelf life. Citric acid and ascorbic acid (vitamin C, ascorbates, E300-4) are natural antioxidants added to a number of foods and they are safe, but synthetic additives such as BHA and BHT (E320-21) may not be.

Alum, an aluminium compound, is used in brands of many pickles to increase crispiness and is also found in some antacids and baking powder. Aluminium (see page 99) has no place in human nutrition.

Nitrates (Nitrites, E249-252) are a type of preservative added to processed meats, such as hot dogs, bacon and ham. Avoid any products containing sodium nitrate or other nitrates.

Monosodium glutamate (MSG or 621) is added to many manufactured foods as a flavour enhancer. It is an unnecessary source of additional sodium in the diet and can cause allergic reactions. Other flavour enhancers and preservatives to avoid include monopotassium glutamate (622) and sodium osinate (631) and benzoic acid and benzoates (E210-9) found in soft drinks, beer and salad creams.

Emulsifiers, stabilisers and thickeners These are found in sauces, soups, breads, biscuits, cakes, frozen desserts, ice cream, margarine and other spreads, jams, chocolate and milk shakes.

More and more manufacturers are cleaning up their products as people become more concerned about toxins in their food and you will increasingly see 'no artificial sweeteners' or 'no artificial ingredients'. This is helpful, but watch out for hidden fats, salts and sugars and alternative names for foods that aren't very good for you when eaten in excess. Sugar, for example, has lots of different names and they include: sucrose, fructose, dextrose and corn syrup. Sodium is just another name for salt, animal fat is saturated fat, trans fatty acid is another name for hydrogenated fat, and sorbitol, saccharine and aspartame are just alternative names for artificial sweeteners.

If you can't understand a label, though, or there's barely room for all the chemical ingredients, leave the product on the shelf.

Drink pure water

It is estimated that as many as 60,000 different chemicals now contaminate our water supply. Numerous studies have found that fish are changing sex due to gender-bending chemicals polluting Britain's rivers (see page 92).[12] In addition to man-made oestrogens, a 2004 report found traces of Prozac and seven other drugs in the UK water supply.[13]

The standard purification techniques used by most water companies remove the bugs from the water but they do not remove all the dissolved chemicals. In attempts to clean the water, other chemicals are often added included chlorine and aluminium. These chemicals may not only be toxic in their own right, but chlorine may react with organic waste to form compounds which can increase the risk of cancer of the colon, rectum and bladder.

We've already seen how important it is if you want to get pregnant to ensure an adequate intake of fluid. And water is just as vital for detoxification as it replenishes, cleanses, rejuvenates and restores your liver, kidneys and adrenals. In fact, it is perhaps the most important part of any healthy eating and detoxification plan.

The recognition that much of our tap water is contaminated has seen a boom in bottled-water sales. The trouble is that the next bottle of water you drink may be nothing more than tap water that has passed through a filter. So when drinking bottled water choose 'mineral' water, otherwise 'spring' water can be just tap water.

The cheapest and easiest way to ensure the water you are drinking is clean and pure is to purify it in your home with water-filter systems. Water-filter jugs are readily available. Use the filtered water for cooking as well as for hot and cold drinks. But bear in mind that filters can become breeding grounds for bacteria so regularly replace the filter and clean the jug. A good-quality filter should eliminate or greatly reduce the levels of heavy metals such as lead, cadmium and chlorine and remove any adverse tastes, colours and smells in the water.

If you want to go to the next level you can install plumbed-in filters for use in your kitchen sink or you can go for one that is fitted to your mains water system at home.

Alternatively, buy mineral water bottled in glass rather than plastic (see page 95).

Avoid exposure to heavy metals

At home and at work many of us are exposed to heavy metals that may pose a risk to our fertility.[14] The main culprits of which you need to be aware and to which you should limit your exposure are listed below:

Lead Lead is a heavy, toxic metal that is naturally present in the earth, but we get exposure to it from lead pipes and car fumes. Research shows that women who live in lead-polluted areas have a higher level of miscarriage. Toxic lead exposure is also associated with birth defects and delayed development. Lead is damaging to male fertility too. Of all the toxic metals, lead, according to a 1991 study, seems to pose the greatest threat to male fertility. Research shows it can reduce sperm count, increase malformed sperm and make sperm sluggish.[15]
Take action: check if your water supply has lead pipes as lead can leach into the water just by standing in the pipes overnight. If you do have lead pipes allow your tap to run for a minute first thing in the morning and use water from the cold not the hot tap as lead dissolves more easily in hot water. Always use a water filter and you should also contact your environmental health department to test the water for you.

All paint is lead-free today but if you are renovating a house built before 1960, be extra careful when scraping or burning off old paint. Take extra precautions, such as wearing a mask or get a professional to do the work for you.

Try not to live near a busy road because of the exhaust fumes from traffic, but if you do, invest in some net curtains to lessen your exposure to car fumes.

Cadmium Cadmium also negatively affects male and female fertility, according to research. It is an inorganic poison present in tobacco smoke that accumulates in the body and blocks the absorption of vital fertility-enhancing nutrients, such as zinc.[16]
Take action: your best course of action is simple: stop smoking and avoid passive smoking.

Aluminium Studies have found that aluminium can also seriously compromise nutritional status and therefore impact on your fertility. The main sources of aluminium are antacids, deodorants, antiperspirants, anti-caking ingredients found in dried milk, aluminium cookware, soft drink cans and foil.[17]
Take action: buy aluminium-free deodorants at health shops.

If you are taking indigestion tablets visit a nutritionist or your doctor to have the cause of the problem investigated.

Throw out all aluminium pans and buy cast iron, enamel, glass and stainless steel and avoid soft drinks in aluminium cans because it can leach into the drinks.

Mercury Mercury is a heavy, toxic metal that now contaminates the air, soil, and water in many parts of the world. Traces of mercury can be found in pesticides, dental fillings and certain fish. The saying 'mad as a hatter' came about because hatters used to polish top hats with mercury, and many of them were poisoned by it.

Mercury is extremely toxic, and studies show it can affect fertility. This may be because the metal accumulates in the pituitary gland, which is vital for stimulating the production of sex hormones, and also because, according to experiments on mice in 1983, it appears to build up in the ovaries themselves. Other research links mercury with painful and irregular periods, reduced fertility rates and premature birth.[18]

Mercury is implicated in miscarriage for workers who are exposed to it in their profession, such as dentists and factory workers who deal with mercury compounds. Women dentists have a higher rate of miscarriage, and female dental assistants who are exposed to mercury through the amalgam fillings they handle have been found to be less fertile than female dentists who do not come into contact with the metal. Recent research urges for the connection between mercury exposure and infertility in both men and women to be further investigated.[19]

If the fillings in your teeth are dark grey or silver, they contain mercury and other metals mixed together into what is called a dental amalgam. Unfortunately, mercury is poisonous, and vapours leach out of our fillings and into the body all the time, especially when we drink something hot like tea or coffee, when we brush our teeth and when we chew gum.

A study of several hundred research papers and clinical reviews suggests that mercury stored in our body may cause a wide variety of symptoms, including allergies, fatigue, mood disorders, flu-like symptoms, menstrual problems, reduced sperm count, ovulation disorders and miscarriage. The use of dental amalgams has been banned in both Sweden and Austria on health grounds. In Japan and Germany, though not prohibited by law, there is a high level of awareness and amalgam fillings are rarely used. In the UK the British Dental Association has not officially accepted that they are a health hazard but a handful of private dentists are willing to help patients get rid of them.

Take action: if you need new fillings ask your dentist for alternatives to amalgam. If you already have amalgams ask your dentist to test for signs of mercury leakage. You may want to consider having any amalgam fillings replaced but unless there are signs that mercury is leaking from them it is better to leave them alone in the pre-conception period as replacing fillings can sometimes release dormant mercury. My advice is to have any necessary dental work done before the three-month pre-conception period and to avoid dental X-rays, fillings and anaesthetics once you are trying to get pregnant. You could be a few weeks pregnant before you know you are and you don't want to risk any exposure to mercury, unless it is an emergency.

Avoid shark, swordfish and marlin as these fish can contain higher levels of mercury. Limit tuna intake to either two fresh tuna steaks a week or four medium tins.

Copper Copper is an essential mineral but it can become toxic if you are exposed to high levels. Your body absorbs copper from water pipes, contraceptive coils, swimming pools and jewellery. Copper levels also increase after hormonal treatments such as fertility drugs. The main issue with copper is that if levels are too high they can deplete zinc levels as the two minerals are antagonistic. Zinc deficiency is a contributing factor to infertility so it is important to keep your copper levels in check.
Take action: avoid copper jewellery when you are trying to conceive. If a mineral test shows that your copper levels are high and zinc low, you need to supplement with extra zinc and establish the source of the copper.

Toxins indoors
Some experts believe that indoor air pollution in homes, offices and other buildings is one of the most serious potential environmental risks to health and fertility. And I'm not just talking about leaking gas fumes or cheap paint, but about the new substances and equipment that have found our way into our homes and lifestyles in the last 50 years due to developments in the building, decorating, carpet, furniture and technological industries.

New carpets, paints and decorating If you're trying to get pregnant you need to take extra special care when decorating your home. Solvent-based paints and white spirits release gases into the air that can linger for weeks after the decorating has finished. In addition, new carpets often contain a chemical preservative called formaldehyde which can irritate the mucus lining of the eyes, nose and throat. An American study of women with a high incidence of unexplained infertility showed them to have high levels of two chemicals found in carpets, leather upholstery and wood preservatives.[20]

The biggest culprits are called VOCs (volatile organic compounds) found in ordinary building and furnishing materials in most homes, including plywood, adhesives, paints, carpets, finishes, synthetic fabrics, household cleaning materials and wood panelling. The most common VOCs are benzenes and formaldehyde.
Take action: when you decorate buy solvent-free paint, take regular fresh air breaks and ventilate the room well before and after. If you need to strip off old paint use a mask and gloves as it may contain lead.

When it comes to furniture and flooring bear in mind that carpets are a major source of poisonous VOCs, especially when new, so if possible allow them to outgas a few days outside your home after they have been delivered. The same applies to furniture, sofa and chairs. Consider having wooden floors and rugs in your home rather than carpet, but if you must have carpet, choose some with latex-free backing and ensure it is nailed rather than glued to the floor.

To avoid unnecessary exposure or risks to your fertility I strongly advise that you do any carpeting, DIY, decorating, furnishing or flooring at least four months before trying for a baby.

Household chemicals Research at Groningen University in the Netherlands commissioned by Greenpeace and WWF (formerly the World Wildlife Fund), reported in 2005, found that every one of the newborn babies monitored had a cocktail of at least five poisonous chemicals in their blood with some babies having as many as 14. These chemicals – found in everyday objects such as soap, cosmetics, cling film, tin cans, toothpaste, baby bottles, furniture, cleaning products and non-stick pans – have been linked to cancer, birth defects and genital abnormalities. They are also being linked to a sharp drop in sperm counts.[21]

Take action: to minimise the chemicals you use in your home such as polish, bleach, detergents and air fresheners, try some of the following instead.

~ Save yourself from exposure to toxic ammonia which can cause irritation of the eyes and respiratory tract, and burn your skin. Mix equal amounts of distilled white or apple cider vinegar and water in a spray bottle. Squirt on windows and wipe with recycled newspapers for a streak-free super shine.

~ A dab of vinegar on a damp cloth is also great for unvarnished wood and when it comes to carpets regular steam cleaning is best as it kills dust mites and bacteria. Make your own deodoriser using a couple of drops of essential oil with baking soda. Sprinkle on carpet, leave for 15 minutes, then vacuum.

~ Put up a detector to protect your family from carbon monoxide exposure. Carbon monoxide starves the body and brain of oxygen and can be fatal. First symptoms include sleepiness, headache, dizziness, flushed skin and disorientation. All homes with gas appliances or heaters should install carbon monoxide detectors, available in most hardware and home-improvement stores or online.

~ Bathroom cleaning sprays produce a fine mist of chemicals that are easily inhaled and can trigger breathing problems. Use two parts water to one part vinegar instead.

~ Instead of chemical-rich floor cleaning products use one cup of vinegar added to a bucket of hot water.

~ Use soap-based or non-biological cleaning products instead of poisonous detergent. While detergents seem safe, they are petrochemical-based products responsible for more household poisonings than any other substance. Soap, on the other hand, is made from natural oils and minerals and has been safely used for centuries. Natural and organic soap-based products can be found in natural food stores and online.

~ Toilet cleaners often contain harsh detergents that are easily absorbed through the skin, causing nausea and irritation of the eye, skin and throat. Many also contain phenol, a suspected cancer-causing agent.

~ Try using a diluted vegetable-based dishwashing liquid.

~ Most air fresheners work by using nerve-deadening agents to stop you detecting smells. They are also one of the most concentrated sources of poison in the home and studies have shown that people who use them have more headaches and skin allergies. You can make your own by adding 10 drops of essential oil to 200g baking soda and placing it in a dish. You can also clear the air with a couple of houseplants. In addition to being beautiful to look at, houseplants also freshen the air by absorbing the carbon dioxide we exhale and releasing the oxygen that is vital for us to breathe. Some plants, such as the popular spider plant, also remove some air pollutants. NASA research has shown that the following plants can help to extract fumes, chemicals and smoke from the air: peace lilies, dwarf banana plants, spider plants, weeping figs, geraniums and chrysanthemums.

Toiletries and cosmetics Many perfumes and scented products contain worrying chemicals so always read labels. Be especially wary of the aluminium in deodorants. Most firms keep their ingredients secret, writing 'parfum' on the label instead so you have no idea what you are spraying onto your body.

Take action: be careful when choosing make-up and moisturisers, etc. as chemicals can get into your skin and be absorbed into the bloodstream. Explore your local health store or reputable online health sites and see what natural alternatives are out there.

Tampons, especially super-absorbent ones may dry out the vagina – making the transfer of toxins into the vagina easier. Best to use towels instead and if you do use tampons make sure you change them every four hours. Some studies have found that the only tampons that do not produce toxins are those that are 100 per cent cotton.

Many commercial bath products contain detergents and artificial fragrances that can be irritating to sensitive areas. You can have a luxurious relaxing bath by adding natural substances to warm bathwater, such as fragrant dried or fresh herbs (try lavender, rosemary, or peppermint), aromatherapy oils or 1 cup Epsom salts. For bubbles, use a natural or organic soap, available in natural food stores and online.

Hair treatments Studies have found that very high doses of the chemicals in hair dyes could cause problems.[22]

Take action: it might be a good idea to avoid colouring your hair or using hair processes and treatments that involve scalp contact when you are trying to get pregnant (and if you are pregnant to wait until you are at least 12 weeks). Highlighting your hair, rather than dyeing it completely, is a good option, as the chemicals are only absorbed by your hair and don't come into contact with your scalp. There are also safe alternatives to chemical dyes, such as henna, which are worth exploring.

Radiation Modern homes are full of devices that emit electromagnetic radiation, including radios, mobiles, electric blankets and microwave ovens. There is also concern about radiation from outside the home in power lines and pylons. Studies have looked at the association with electrical radiation and infertility and cot death but the evidence is still hotly debated.[23]

Take action: until more is known, as a simple precaution it might be worth keeping radiation to a minimum in the areas you spend most of your time in at home – the bedroom, kitchen and living room.

Mobile phones and VDUs You may want to limit mobile phone use and the amount of television you watch. Studies on animals exposed to mobile phone and VDU radiation suggest there could be an increased risk of miscarriage. Recent research has shown that the use of mobile phones by men decreases sperm motility and sperm count and increases the number of abnormal sperm. The negative change in sperm was connected to the daily exposure of mobile phone use and was independent of the initial semen quality.[24]

Take action: much more research needs to be done but, for now, the fact that a link is suspected should be enough incentive to cut down daily use of mobiles, televisions, electrical appliances and computers.

~ Keep use of your mobile to a minimum and use a landline wherever possible. Buy a separate mike so that the handset is not next to your head. If you carry a mobile keep the handset as far away from your body as possible. Your partner should avoid carrying it in his trouser pockets, or on a belt near his testes as this increases the risk of electromagnetic radiation emitted by the handset or the heat it generates.

~ Position electrical alarm clocks and radios so that they are not right next to your head when you are sleeping.

~ Keep a good distance from televisions and VDUs, limiting use to no more than four hours a day if possible.

Electrical appliances Avoid electrical appliances with PCBs (polychlorinated biphenyls, a group of man-made chemicals). They were once widely used in electrical equipment, in industrial processes, and in the manufacture and recycling of carbonless copy paper until research revealed that they pose risks to human health, wildlife and the natural environment. The government banned the production of PCBs in the 1970s but PCB contamination remains widespread in the environment today because of improper disposal of products containing the chemicals and by-products of the processes used to make them. Men exposed to high levels of PCBs were found to be 60 per cent more likely to have sperm with DNA damage.[25]

Microwave ovens The majority of modern homes have microwave ovens which heat food using high-frequency electromagnetic waves. There are concerns not just about radiation leaking into food but about the food being inherently damaged by the way it is being cooked. For instance, studies on microwaved carrots and broccoli show that their molecular structure is deformed whereas in normal cooking it is not.[26] All this means that microwave cooking may encourage the production of free radicals.

More research needs to be done but at a time when you are trying to get pregnant it makes sense to avoid anything that could be a potential threat to your fertility. *Take action:* if you must use a microwave, never stand directly in front of it when it is on, have it checked regularly for leaks and, best of all, consider whether you really need it.

Toxins in the workplace

In 1997 the *Lancet* published a list of occupations and agents that may be toxic to fertility.[27] More recently other studies have confirmed links between particular jobs and reduced fertility in both men and women. Here are their conclusions:[28]

Taxi and lorry drivers Studies show that long hours spent sitting and driving can result in lower than normal sperm count or abnormal sperm.[29]

Welders, bakers, cooks and fire fighters Any job that exposes a man to intense heat can result in reduced quality and quantity of sperm. In addition, fire fighters are exposed to a large variety of chemicals which can affect their health and fertility.[30]

Painters, cleaners and lab workers Exposure to solvents and toxins can reduce fertility in both men and women, although right now the evidence suggests it may have more of a damaging effect in women.[31]

Farmers Agricultural workers exposed to pesticides and other chemicals have been shown to have low sperm counts.[32]

Health care workers, doctors, vets and dentists The fertility of both men and women who are regularly exposed to anaesthetic gases, ethylene oxide, cytostatic drugs, mercury and x-rays is at risk. Men who are exposed to x-rays through work are especially likely to have reduced sperm counts.[33] Also, dentists and their assistants may experience problems due to mercury amalgam fillings (see page 100).

Painters, decorators and printers As outlined in the decorating section above, regular exposure to solvents and pigments can affect male and female fertility.

Traffic wardens Anyone exposed to traffic fumes on a regular basis from traffic wardens to garage attendants and mechanics may be at risk of diesel toxicity.[34]

Workers in manufacturing industries Women whose work involves contact with formaldehyde may experience reduced fertility. Those especially at risk include hospital staff as well as workers in the plastics, paints, foam, resin and furniture manufacturing industries. In addition, the chemical carbon disulphide in several manufacturing processes, such as the production of plastics, has been linked to sexual dysfunction in both men and women and glycol ethers used by electronics manufacturing have also been shown to reduce sperm count.[35]

Gardeners Many pesticides and herbicides, including DDT, lindane and paraquat, are known reproductive toxins that can play havoc with hormonal health and lower sperm count. People working in gardens, parks, plant nurseries and farms are at risk.[36]

Dry cleaners and manicurists Women who work in nail salons or dry cleaners while pregnant are at an increased risk of having a child with learning difficulties. One study showed that exposure to solvents in the workplace during pregnancy resulted in children with shorter attention spans and lower IQ.[37] The researchers stress that it does not apply to women who are occasionally visiting a nail salon but it would still be worth keeping visits to an absolute minimum during pregnancy and avoiding exposure during the first 12 weeks during the period of maximum cell division.

Hair stylists Women who've spent many years in daily contact with hair dye chemicals do appear to have a slightly higher risk of having a miscarriage. This is thought to be due to regular contact with chemicals in dyes called teratogens, which can cause birth defects and increase the risk of miscarriage.

Workers in high-stress occupations Stress is a known inhibitor of fertility (see page 63) and there could be a link between any high-stress occupation and an increased risk of miscarriage, according to recent research.[38]

In addition to toxic exposure and the stress of a demanding job, there are other work-related fertility hazards for women. A 2003 study showed that shift work may pose a threat to fertility, and other studies confirm this.[39] Night workers, pilots and air stewardesses may also have problems conceiving because lack of daylight or time differences can interfere with their menstrual cycle and ovulation. In men the stress that unusual hours put on the body can also damage their health and fertility.[40] Noise pollution, long working hours and jobs with high public contact have also been shown to cause problems in pregnancy.[41]

Computers Computers produce a range of electromagnetic radiation frequencies, but not enough is known about the impact of extended use on health and fertility.

Recent research suggests that work with computers is safe but some believe it may pose a risk. One study found that women who spent more than 20 hours a week in front of a computer screen had twice the number of miscarriages than non VDU users.[42] Another showed that spending up to six hours a day at a computer increased the risk of miscarriage, premature birth or stillbirth.[43]

Some scientists suggest that men may be more at risk than women from the effects of VDUs because their genitals being external are not so well protected but again research is still preliminary and no firm conclusions have been drawn. There are indications, however, that excessive use of laptops may be most detrimental. The problem comes from two factors – the laptop itself generates heat but having the legs closed to balance the laptop also raises the temperature. Using healthy volunteers, researchers found that the temperature in that area rose by 2.1°C even when the men simply sat with their thighs together without a laptop. With the laptop, the temperature rose by up to 2.8°C. Increases in temperature around the testes by just 1 degree can decrease fertility by 40 per cent.[44]

It seems obvious to me that radiation may not be the only reason for the increased risk of infertility in men and women who routinely use VDUs. The length of time sitting at the computer doing repetitive or stressful work under pressure could add to the problem as regular exercise and stress management are important fertility-boosting factors.

Take action: if you must work at a computer for extended periods there are certain precautions you should take:

~ To reduce your risk of VDU radiation keep the time spent on the VDU to a minimum – around four or five hours. If you have to work at your computer all day, have breaks every 30 minutes to get up and stretch or better still have a breath of fresh air.

~ Don't put laptops on your lap; use a table instead.

~ Switch the VDU off when you aren't using it, rather than using the screensaver.

~ An ioniser on top of your desk might help as can an amethyst crystal which is said to help absorb static.

~ Put natural fibre, for example wool, carpets or wooden floors under your VDU and have it earthed.

~ To check for hazardous frequencies leave a vase of flowers next to your VDU and another a few feet away and see which wilts faster. If the flowers are degrading quicker when next to the computer then place some plants like spider plants, ficus and the cactus mentioned below to help offset the effect.

~ According to the Institut de Recherches en Géobiologie at Chardonne in Switzerland a cactus called *Cereus peruvianus* can help to absorb VDU radiation.

OCCUPATIONAL RISKS FOR YOUR PARTNER Many occupations, as listed above, carry risks in terms of male fertility. Your partner should:

~ avoid tight trousers or underpants, especially nylon ones

~ shower his genitals with cold water to lower their temperature and improve circulation

~ avoid vigorous sports and long-distance cycling in the pre-conception period

~ limit computer and mobile phone use.

YOUR RIGHTS If after reading the section on occupational hazards you think your work may be exposing you to unnecessary health risks there are many things you can do, whether you are male or female. For advice about occupational health risks contact your trade organisation or health and safety officer. If your employer isn't interested, talk to your union, if you have one or a lawyer – you have the legal right to ask your employer for a written assessment of any possible risks to your health and fertility. If risks are identified your employer or company is then legally obliged to take measures to protect you.

DON'T GO OVERBOARD

No fertility-boosting plan is complete without taking into account the effect of hormonally active agents in the environment and in your workplace – whether they are swallowed or inhaled, voluntarily or involuntarily. Taking measures to avoid toxins in the food you eat and the environment you live and work in can help to protect you from possible hormonal disturbance and to reduce the toxic load.

But does this mean you must never have unfiltered water, wear perfume or spend time working on the computer again? No, not at all. As with your fertility-boosting diet remember the 80:20 rule because it applies here as well, i.e. if you get it right 80 per cent of the time you are doing brilliantly. You still have to live in the real world and the odd slip-up is fine.

Healthy eating, regular exercise and commonsense precautions to avoid over-exposure to toxins as much as possible are, more often than not, sufficient to reduce the risk of toxic overload in terms of your fertility. So don't go overboard. Remember you are trying to do all you can to boost your chances of having a healthy baby and that means not stressing yourself out over anything – including extreme and unsustainable lifestyle changes.

CHECKLIST FOR AVOIDING OCCUPATIONAL AND ENVIRONMENTAL TOXINS

~ Eat only organic food or as much as you can.

~ Wash all your fruit and vegetables thoroughly before use.

~ Filter your water.

~ Reduce your intake of fatty animal products (xenoestrogens love fat!).

~ Don't wrap or heat food in plastic or cling film.

~ Refuse mercury fillings.

~ Avoid aluminium kitchenware, foil and foods.

~ Avoid cigarette smoke and heavily lead-polluted air; don't stand around in heavy traffic and close car windows when going through tunnels.

~ Check ingredients in toiletries, cosmetics, deodorants, perfumes, air fresheners and cleaning products and use natural ones instead.

~ Regularly check what toxins you may be exposed to at work or in the house or garden.

~ Limit computer and mobile phone time or take regular breaks.

~ See green: at least once a day, take a stroll in a park or green place. Trees and plants give out energising oxygen. It's also a good idea to have plants in your home and workplace.

step five
screening
for infections

As well as making positive changes to your diet and lifestyle, it's a good idea to get checked for infections, especially if you have been trying to conceive for a while without success or have had a previous miscarriage. In my clinics, patients always have a pre-conception check-up that includes discussion of the following.

YOUR MEDICAL HISTORY

Your pre-conception check-up is the best time to talk through any health concerns or worries you may have, so it might be worth preparing a list of questions. During your check-up you and your partner will be asked about your health and lifestyle, eating and exercise habits and any possible exposure to environmental hazards at home or at work.

This is also the time to mention any medications, supplements or herbs you are taking to check that they are safe to take during pregnancy and that they do not affect your fertility. Questions will be asked about what kind of contraception you are or have been using (see Step 6) and whether you've had any ovulation or menstruation problems, terminations, miscarriages, delivery complications and the like. If you have had problems in the past with menstruation or a pelvic infection, tests or a referral to a gynaecologist may be recommended. If you have a condition such as polycystic ovaries, you can start treating the problem now and increase your odds of a healthy pregnancy. (Step 7 looks at the impact of any common gynaecological and long-term health problems on your future pregnancy.)

There are some infections that can impact on your fertility or increase the risk of a miscarriage while others do not stop you getting or staying pregnant but need to be eliminated or prevented because they can have an effect on the baby once you are pregnant.

TEST FOR INFECTIONS

To increase your chances of a successful pregnancy, it's extremely important for you to discuss the possibility of sexually transmitted infections (STDs or STIs) with your doctor. There are also a number of genito-urinary infections (GUIs) (affecting the urinary tract and genitals) that can stop you getting pregnant or cause miscarriages and because many of them don't have noticeable symptoms you may not even know that you have them.

If you feel uncomfortable talking to your doctor you can go to a specialist GUM (genito-urinary medicine) clinic without a referral; they will test for the possibility of STDs but may not test for all of the infections that can affect fertility.

Getting tested for potentially fertility-robbing infections is so important for your fertility and the health of your future baby that Step 5 of my fertility-boosting plan is devoted to the most common infections that inhibit fertility and what you need to know about them.

FERTILITY-ROBBING INFECTIONS

As many vaginal or pelvic infections can increase your risk of infertility, miscarriage and pre-term delivery as well as infection in your future child I can't stress enough how important it is for you to have a GUI screening during the pre-conception period, especially if you notice any of the following symptoms:

~ itching, soreness, tenderness or pain in the vagina
~ any abnormal vaginal discharge, for example, unusual smelling or staining
~ pain on urinating
~ low abdominal pain
~ discomfort during intercourse
~ abnormal bleeding
~ lumps or ulcers in genital area
~ genital problems in your partners – past and present.

Common symptoms of sexually transmitted diseases in men include:

~ discharge from the penis
~ soreness or ulcers in genital area
~ frequent urge to urinate and pain when passing urine (urethritis)
~ swollen glands in the groin
~ painful testes or prostate gland.

The GUI screening for men I use in my clinics involves a urine test, the taking of a urethral swab or prostatic massage and a semen culture.

Listed below are those infections most likely to play havoc with your fertility and which both you and/or your partner need to be screened for.

PELVIC INFLAMMATORY DISEASE (PID)

PID is an umbrella term for any inflammation of the organs in the pelvis. It is normally caused by an infection which can affect any of the reproductive organs, including the womb, ovaries, fallopian tubes, cervix, womb lining and/or vagina. PID is sexually transmitted and is typically caused by anaerobic bacteria and chlamydia infection (see page 113), but it can be caused by infections such as gonorrhoea (see page 114) or result from a surgical procedure such as implantation of a contraceptive coil. The symptoms of PID are usually pelvic pain, vaginal discharge and a fever although PID can often be silent and may cause mild abdominal pain or bleeding during intercourse or prolonged bleeding. Sometimes there are no symptoms at all.

The infertile acid mucus that is produced most of the month acts as a barrier not only to sperm but to most other organisms. Around ovulation it becomes 'fertile mucus' which is more alkaline and stretchy, allowing the passage of the sperm but opening the floodgates to negative organisms. Some organisms also attach themselves to sperm, 'hitching a ride' further into the body.[1] Parasites like trichomonads can also carry unwanted organisms with them when they move from the vagina to the fallopian tubes so it is possible to have more than one infection at the same time.

How does it affect fertility?

Eventually, as the infection subsides the organs become scarred and the fallopian tubes become blocked making fertilisation unlikely if not impossible. Even if the fallopian tubes are merely distorted a fertilised egg may still have difficulty travelling to the womb and an ectopic pregnancy is more likely to occur. Studies suggest that as many as 15 per cent of women have had symptoms of PID by the age of 30. After one attack, 80 per cent of sufferers will have irregular or heavy periods and 40 per cent will suffer pain after intercourse. A further 20 per cent will experience chronic pelvic pain and 13 per cent will have problems conceiving. In addition, the risk of an ectopic pregnancy (when a fertilised egg implants in the fallopian tube) is seven times greater in women who have had one attack of PID. After a second attack infertility rises to 35 per cent and after a third 75 per cent of women are infertile because their fallopian tubes are blocked and scarred.[2]

Testing This is done with a vaginal swab.

Treatment PID should be treated immediately it is diagnosed because it is a serious threat to your fertility. Any woman who has symptoms must go to her doctor without delay because if PID is severe it can be life-threatening. Antibiotics can be prescribed to treat the infection but will not be able to reverse any scarring that has taken place, so the earlier antibiotics are taken the better.

CHLAMYDIA

Chlamydia, often described as an 'infertility time bomb' is a bacterial infection that can cause reproductive problems for women who contract it prior to and during pregnancy. The Royal College of Physicians estimates that this is the most common sexually transmitted disease of them all and the most common cause of PID in the world.[3] The UK government is considering the idea of national screening for chlamydia but there are many issues that need to be resolved before this comes into force.

Chlamydia occurs most frequently in people under the age of 25. The most frightening thing about it is that up to 70 per cent of women don't realise that they have it because there are no noticeable symptoms, although a minority report burning on urination and vaginal discharge. In men, chlamydia can cause symptoms of urethritis (an infection of the urethra) such as a burning sensation on passing urine. If men don't get treated they can pass the infection on to their partners.[4]

How does if affect fertility?

Untreated, chlamydia can spread to the upper genital tract (womb, fallopian tubes and ovaries), resulting in PID (see page 112) and the possibility of ectopic pregnancy or infertility. It can also cause inflammation of the cervix, resulting in temporary infertility by affecting the cervical mucus.

Up to 10 per cent of pregnant women may have chlamydia. Untreated, they may face an increased risk of miscarriage and premature rupture of the membranes (the fluid bag surrounding the baby). A study from the National Institute of Child Health and Human Development suggested that pregnant women with chlamydia have a two- to three-fold increased risk of pre-term delivery.[5]

Men with chlamydia may also have an infection in the testes and epididymis, which can decrease the quality of their sperm. It is thought to affect one in ten men, damaging not only the quality and quantity of sperm but also sperm DNA (see page 47), making it more difficult for the sperm to fertilise the egg. Also, men can be passing chlamydia on to their partners, without even knowing they have it themselves.

Testing Testing for chlamydia can be done with a urine sample or vaginal swab.

Treatment Chlamydia can be treated easily with antibiotics. Both partners should be screened and, if necessary, treated because the infection can be passed back and forth between you. Most people do not become immune to chlamydia so it is quite possible to become re-infected with the disease by another sexual partner.[6] If you are pregnant and have a chlamydia infection it is very important to have it treated right away as it can be passed on to your baby, possibly causing severe eye damage and lung infections.

TAKING ANTIBIOTICS When you take an antibiotic to treat an infection, it will eliminate the healthy as well as the unhealthy bacteria which could leave you susceptible to an attack of thrush (yeast overgrowth). So alongside the antibiotics you should take a good probiotic supplement containing different strains of beneficial bacteria for three months (don't use the probiotic drinks which can be loaded with sugar and will 'feed' the yeast). You can also get special probiotic pessaries to insert vaginally which you would use with the oral probiotic, but don't use these once you are trying to conceive. Also, if you have been on the Pill in the last year it is worth taking a probiotic for three months as it can upset the balance of bacteria.

GONORRHOEA

Gonorrhoea is a common bacterial infection that causes reproductive problems like those caused by chlamydia. It has no symptoms in infected women, though some experience a yellow vaginal discharge, burning on urination or abdominal pain. Men with gonorrhoea may suffer from a penile discharge and/or urethritis (an infection of the urethra).

How does it affect fertility?
In women gonorrhoea can cause PID by spreading up through the cervix and infecting the womb and fallopian tubes which can lead to infertility. Pregnant women with untreated gonorrhoea are at increased risk of miscarriage, premature delivery, and premature rupture of the membranes. Their babies frequently contract this STI during vaginal delivery. Infected babies sometimes develop serious eye and joint infections and, less commonly, life-threatening blood infections, which are treated with antibiotics. Untreated, gonorrhoea in men can spread to all the sexual organs and affect fertility.[7]

Testing Testing for gonorrhoea is done with a urine sample or a vaginal swab.

Treatment Gonorrhoea is treated with antibiotics. Although it is slowly being eradicated, both you and your partner should be screened and if necessary treated.

BACTERIAL VAGINOSIS (GARDNERELLA)

Most bacteria living in your vagina need oxygen to survive and are aerobic but a minority are anaerobic, preferring lower levels of oxygen. Bacterial imbalance occurs when anaerobes outnumber the protective, aerobic bacteria and this causes bacterial vaginosis (BV), affecting about 16 per cent of pregnant women. When BV is present the normal – slightly acidic – quality of the vagina becomes more alkaline.

Doctors don't know for sure how a woman gets BV, though it appears more common in women who have new or multiple sexual partners. It is not classed as a sexually transmitted disease and men do not usually get it, so it is thought that semen can change the pH of the vagina. Women with BV can experience vaginal discharge that has an unpleasant odour, burning on urination and genital itching.

How does it affect fertility?

BV can impact on your fertility by affecting the quality of your cervical mucus. It could also increase the risk of a miscarriage, so it is best to be treated before you start trying to conceive. It is very common and accounts for up to 50 per cent of all vaginal infections. Studies suggest that BV may double a woman's chances of pre-term delivery.[8]

Testing Testing for BV is with a vaginal swab.

Treatment The treatment for BV usually takes the form of drugs, such as antibiotics or an antimicrobial, e.g. metronidazole that eliminates anaerobic bacteria. It is important that you have conventional medical treatment for BV but then you should work on prevention. Because BV tends to proliferate when the balance between healthy and unhealthy bacteria in the body changes it is important that your levels of beneficial bacteria are good. Research has shown that one of the beneficial bacteria, lactobacillus, is toxic to Gardnerella vaginalis (the main cause of bacterial vaginosis).[9] You should take a good probiotic to improve the levels of good bacteria in your body and use a few drops of tea tree oil (which is antimicrobial) in your bath.

TRICHOMONAS

Trichomoniasis is a parasitic infection that causes yellow-green foul-smelling vaginal discharge, genital itching and redness and pain during intercourse and urination. Men with trichomoniasis are often symptom-free, although they can suffer from a sore glans (the tip of the penis) and urethritis and pain on urination.

How does it affect fertility?

Trichomoniasis tends not to cause pelvic infection in women, but it can inhibit fertility by interfering with the quality of cervical mucus. Untreated, trichomoniasis may also increase the risk of premature rupture of the membranes and pre-term delivery.[10]

Testing Testing for this infection is with a vaginal swab. For men, this will include a visual examination of the penis and a sample of discharge from the urethra.

Treatment Trichomoniasis can usually be treated with metronidazole. Because it is sexually transmitted both partners should be treated.[11]

CYTOMEGALOVIRUS (CMV)

CMV belongs to the same family of viral infections that causes genital herpes, chicken pox and shingles. CMV is fairly common and may cause a mild flu-like illness until the infection passes.

CMV during pregnancy is linked with an increased risk of miscarriage and pre-term labour, physical and metal retardation in the baby, hearing problems, jaundice and chest and eye infections.[12] It is estimated that 3,000 babies are infected each year in the UK, with 300 suffering a subsequent handicap. To reduce your risk of infection with CMV make sure you avoid animals or humans who are clearly sick. CMV is also excreted in saliva and urine so pregnant women and women trying to conceive should avoid kissing and cuddling young children as the incidence is highest in the first years of life.

How does it affect fertility?

CMV may affect a man by reducing his sperm count.[13] It will not affect your fertility but can be passed from you to your baby during pregnancy and the earlier in your pregnancy the infection occurs the more serious the risk (see above).

Testing CMV is detected using a blood test.

Treatment There is no treatment for CMV just prevention as mentioned above.

MYCOPLASMA AND UREAPLASMA

These organisms are commonly found in the GUI tracts of both men and women but are found more in couples who are having problems getting pregnant. Symptoms include burning on urination, constant feeling of need to urinate, vaginal itching, odour or discharge.

How does it affect fertility?

Research suggests that mycoplasma may increase the percentage of abnormal sperm and may affect sperm by lowering the amount of zinc and fructose in sperm. Zinc is crucial for healthy sperm and fructose is the sugar that the sperm use as fuel for the journey through the vagina to the egg.[14]

Studies have also linked these microbes with an increased risk of miscarriage so if you have had an unexplained miscarriage or have used the Pill for many years (mycoplasma proliferates when the Pill is used) testing for mycoplasma and ureaplasma is strongly advised.[15] If a pregnant woman has a ureaplasma infection she can pass it on to her baby and increase their risk of asthma.[16]

Testing For women a vaginal swab is used to test for these organisms and for men a sample of cells is collected from the entrance of the urethra and tested along with a urine sample.

Treatment Antibiotics are used to treat mycoplasma and ureaplasma in both men and women.

CANDIDA ALBICANS

Also called thrush, this common yeast infection affects many women whether they are sexually active or not. Candida is a yeast present in the vagina with which problems can occur if it multiplies, upsetting the natural balance of bacteria. This tends to happen when blood sugar levels are too high and also after a course of antibiotics which can destroy many good bacteria along with the unhealthy ones, giving candida an opportunity to thrive. It can cause a white, lumpy discharge and intense itching or burning. Intercourse can be painful because the vagina is sore.

Previous use of the Pill can also cause problems with candida.[17]

Candida can affect you getting pregnant by putting you off intercourse because having sex is just too painful. It can also make the vaginal environment more hostile to sperm. It is important to clear up any infection before you conceive or during pregnancy as your baby may catch the infection from the birth canal during delivery. Infection in the baby can lead to nappy rash and a sore mouth, which can cause feeding difficulties. Thrush is extremely common in pregnancy, and may affect up to one in four women because a pregnant woman's vaginal secretions favour the growth of yeast. Candida in men can cause soreness or itching of the penis.

Anti-fungal treatments are usually effective at treating thrush and can be used safely during the pre-conception period. But it is better to treat it naturally when you can. Probiotic supplements, containing Lactobacilli and Bifidobacterium are beneficial. Garlic is another natural anti-fungal remedy and one of the best supplements is aged garlic. To prevent the likelihood of other attacks avoid wearing tight jeans, synthetic underwear or panty liners unnecessarily. Modern low-temperature washing machine cycles don't always kill candida spores and re-infection can occur from your own underwear so hot iron the gussets on your underwear or use a hotter wash. You should also eliminate foods high in sugar, such as sweets, cakes, refined foods and drinks and alcohol.

Candida also exists naturally in the intestines. When you are in good health it remains a single-cell organism kept under control by beneficial bacteria and your immune system. If you are under stress or run down the yeast can change form and become 'mycelial' which has root-like growths. These roots can then penetrate the walls of the digestive system causing an infection of candida throughout the body, known as 'candidiasis'. If you have candidiasis it causes an immune response (because your body is trying to fight the infection) and this can be picked up in a simple test (see page 218). Symptoms of candidiasis include persistent vaginal thrush, bloating and flatulence, cravings for sugar and bread, getting tipsy on a small amount of alcohol, brain fog, athlete's foot and fungal toe. Candidiasis should be treated because it affects your general health and, in turn, fertility.

INFECTIONS THAT CAN CAUSE A PROBLEM ONCE YOU ARE PREGNANT

The following infections won't affect fertility but can impact on the baby during pregnancy.

SYPHILIS

Syphilis is a dangerous STD (sexually transmitted disease) caused by a bacterium, which can cross the placenta and infect the foetus. Fortunately, the number of new cases in women of child-bearing age has dropped to an all-time low (2,219 cases in 2000) in the UK and USA. Syphilis begins with a hard, painless sore called a chancre in the genital or vaginal area. Untreated, infected individuals develop a rash, fever and other symptoms months later. If still untreated, years later some infected individuals develop devastating damage to many organs that result in heart problems, brain damage, blindness, insanity and death.[18]

Syphilis can be passed on to your baby during pregnancy, so to protect your health and that of your baby it is important to be treated before you start trying for a baby. Without treatment, syphilis during pregnancy can result in foetal or infant death in up to 40 per cent of cases. Some infected infants show no symptoms at birth, but without immediate antibiotic treatment, develop brain damage, blindness, hearing loss, bone and tooth abnormalities and other problems.[19]

Treatment A blood test is used to screen for syphilis. A single dose of penicillin can cure it if a woman has had the infection for less than a year; others will require longer periods of treatment. When a woman is treated by the fourth month of pregnancy, her baby usually will not be harmed. Treatment for men is also with antibiotics.

RUBELLA

German measles contracted in childhood is a mild disease and once infected a person has lifelong immunity. A blood test can tell you whether you are rubella immune or not. The risk of contracting German measles during pregnancy is not to the mother but to the baby. If the mother develops the illness in the first 12 weeks of pregnancy there is a five times greater chance of the baby being miscarried or born with congenital abnormalities.

If you are not immune you may decide to be vaccinated before you become pregnant. If you do, you should wait at least three months before trying to conceive. Your body will need time to eliminate the injected virus, as it's theoretically possible for an unborn child to contract the virus and (as with rubella) suffer birth defects including deafness, encephalitis and heart problems.

Note: all vaccines are best avoided during pregnancy unless there is a definite risk of infection. You would need to take this into account if you are travelling to a country that requires certain vaccinations for entry.

GENITAL HERPES

Genital herpes is caused by the herpes simplex virus. Although for the majority there are few symptoms it can cause tiny, painful ulcers around the vagina and cervix in women and on the penis in men. The virus can remain dormant in a person's nerve cells indefinitely once they are infected, flaring up during times of stress or illness. Usually, herpes can only be transmitted to your partner when you have an attack of the infection with ulcers and blisters. Herpes will not affect your ability to conceive and does not tend to affect your baby during pregnancy. However, an attack near the time of birth could result in your baby catching the infection. A small minority of women with herpes pass it on to their infants during vaginal delivery. The risk is highest (30 to 50 per cent) when the pregnant woman contracts herpes (whether or not she has symptoms) for the first time late in pregnancy. Some infected infants develop skin or mouth sores, which can usually be effectively treated with anti-viral drugs. However, in spite of treatment, the infection sometimes spreads to the brain and internal organs, resulting in brain damage, blindness, mental retardation and even death. If a woman has symptoms of herpes at the time of delivery, a Caesarean section will probably be recommended to protect the baby.[20]

Treatment Doctors usually diagnose herpes by looking at the sores; however, in some cases, they may take a swab of the blisters for testing. Acyclovir and other anti-viral drugs are helpful in shortening attacks but cannot cure the disease completely.

HIV (HUMAN IMMUNODEFICIENCY VIRUS)

HIV is the virus that causes AIDS (acquired immune deficiency syndrome), which can damage the immune system and threaten the lives of mothers and babies. HIV can be transmitted by sexual contact, needle sharing and blood transfusions and by pregnant mothers to their babies. The virus can only be detected several months after it has been acquired because it takes this long for antibodies to appear in the blood.

Your fertility may not be affected by HIV or AIDS but infection has potentially fatal consequences for both you and your unborn child. Babies of mothers infected with HIV may be born with the virus and are likely to develop full-blown AIDS by their second birthday. Breastfeeding mothers with HIV may also transmit the virus to their children.

Treatment The Center for Disease Control and Prevention (CDC) in the USA recommends that all pregnant women be offered counselling and voluntary testing for HIV. Women who learn that they carry the virus can get treatment to help protect their babies. New drug treatments can now reduce to 2 per cent or less the risk of a treated mother passing HIV on to her baby, compared to about 25 per cent of untreated mothers.

INFECTION-FIGHTING FOODS Following my guidelines for diet and supplements is the best way to boost your immune system and prevent infections. You should also eliminate foods that contain yeast and sugar if you have a yeast infection. If you're on antibiotics take a good broad-spectrum probiotic supplement (see page 20). Other foods that may be helpful include:

Cruciferous vegetables: broccoli, cauliflower, cabbage, Brussels sprouts and turnips – all rich in beta carotene (see page 24), vital for the functioning of the immune system and the normal growth of vaginal tissue.

Garlic: nature's foremost immune-enhancing food and also a rich source of selenium. One of the best supplement forms of garlic is aged garlic (available from www.naturalhealthpractice.com).

Oily fish: (see page 22) contain the EFAs for producing immune factors such as white blood cells.

Raw almonds: great source of essential amino acids and EFAs.

Berries: rich in vitamin C for the formation of collagen, making infection less able to spread.

Sunflower seeds: excellent source of vitamin E which helps increase resistance to chlamydia infections.

Eggs: good source of vitamin B; women with vaginal infections are often deficient in B vitamins.

Legumes: great source of zinc which can boost immunity, encourage healing and prevent recurrence of infection.

LISTERIA

This bacterial infection is common in cattle, pigs and poultry and can affect humans with a flu-like illness after exposure, the main symptom being diarrhoea. Listeria can be life threatening in pregnant women and can also be passed from mother to child during pregnancy, although fortunately infection of unborn babies remains rare at around one in 30,000. Listeria infection during pregnancy is linked with miscarriage, stillbirth, pre-term delivery and severe illness in the newborn, such as meningitis.[21]

As well as being common in livestock, listeria is also widespread in the soil and foods with a high listeria risk should be avoided. Pasteurisation usually destroys the bacteria but if food is infected and then refrigerated, listeria will multiply. Foods to avoid in the pre-conception period and during pregnancy include: ripe soft cheese (such as Brie), blue-veined cheese (such as Stilton), goat's or sheep cheese (for example feta), any unpasteurised soft or cream cheese; undercooked meat and ready-to-eat poultry; ready made cook-chill meals; all types of pâté; prepared salads and coleslaw; foods past their sell-by date. Hard cheese is safe, as is cottage cheese.

Finally, because listeria can be passed on through contact with infected animals women should be especially careful when visiting farms or travelling abroad in countries where the incidence of food contamination and infection is high. If listeria is suspected treatment will involve hospitalisation and high-dose antibiotics.

TOXOPLASMOSIS

This food-borne infection is caused by a parasite called Toxoplasma gondii and is found in many animals but the cat is its reproductive host. It can be caught from handling the faeces of cats, eating raw or undercooked meat, unwashed vegetables, unpasteurised dairy products and drinking contaminated water. Toxoplasmosis is a common infection but once you have it you usually become immune. A simple blood test in the pre-conception period will let you know if you carry the antibodies to protect you and your baby from toxoplasmosis.

If a woman gets toxoplasmosis during pregnancy the baby is usually infected in 45 per cent of cases. The risk to the baby is greatest in the first 12 weeks and can cause eye problems, convulsions, blindness, brain damage and hydrocephalus (accumulation of fluid on the brain). Preventative measures should include washing your hands or using gloves to handle cats or kittens and emptying litter trays within 24 hours (before the parasite becomes active). Wash vegetables carefully, don't drink or cook with unpasteurised milk and cook raw meat thoroughly. Gloves should also be worn while gardening.

GROUP B STREPTOCOCCUS (GBS)

This common bacterial infection does not affect fertility but is associated with late miscarriages, stillbirths, premature rupture of the membranes and premature birth. Pregnant women should be treated with antibiotics to prevent the infection spreading to the baby.[22] Testing for GBS with vaginal and rectal swabs is routinely done as part of antenatal care in many countries including USA, Canada and Australia. Often there are no symptoms but GBS can manifest as urinary tract or infections of the womb. It is treated with antibiotics.

POSSIBLE INFECTIONS (OLD AND NEW) IN YOUR PARTNER

Any infection of the urinary tract and prostate that your partner has or had in the past (even if they have all cleared up) may have caused damage and be affecting his fertility now. Mumps could be one of those. Caused by a virus, mumps is not a problem when children are young, but in older boys and men it can lead to inflammation of the testes (orchitis) and can affect fertility later on. Some infections can remain at a very low, sub-clinical level, not causing symptoms but detectable on medical testing. If sperm is infected, even at a mild, symptomless level, it can make all the difference between being able to create a successful pregnancy and not.

The same applies for STDS, like chlamydia and non-specific urethritis (NSU) – an infection of the urinal tract that has been linked with abnormal sperm and low sperm count. Any one of several infections can cause NSU and your partner will need to find out which one via his doctor or a GUI clinic.

INFECTIONS FOR WHICH BOTH PARTNERS SHOULD BE SCREENED

~ Chlamydia

~ Gonorrhoea

~ Bacterial vaginosis (gardnerella vaginalis)

~ Trichomonas

~ Cytomegalovirus (CMV)

~ Mycoplasmas/ureaplasmas

~ Candida albicans

~ Toxoplasmosis

~ Group B streptococcus

~ Mixed anaerobes

~ Syphilis

GUI clinics can test for some of these infections but if you are having problems conceiving or have had a problem with miscarriage, it is worth checking them all.

Don't be tempted to skip this important step in my fertility-boosting plan, thinking it can't happen to you. Infections can happen to anyone at any time, so to avoid unnecessary complications and heartache and to give yourself peace of mind, it is vital that you and your partner are screened for infections in the pre-conception period.

step six
getting the *timing* right

A baby is conceived around the time of ovulation, during your fertile period. There are various ways in which you can judge when you are ovulating. By identifying this fertile period you can make a point of having intercourse to maximise your chances of conceiving. You can also use fertility awareness to help you avoid getting pregnant until you are ready to become a mother.

Recognising your fertility signals is an important part of my fertility-boosting plan and in this section you'll learn how to get the timing right to give yourself the best chance of getting pregnant. Before that, however, it is also important to discuss the issue of contraception – which method is the most suitable while you and your partner prepare for pregnancy and when is the best time to stop using it.

CONTRACEPTION AND FERTILITY

You may be wondering why we're discussing contraception in a book about fertility! While you are getting as fit and as well as you can before trying to conceive, you need to use a form of contraception you can trust but which will also allow your fertility to return quickly when you stop using it.

THE PILL

I'm often asked by women using the oral contraceptive pill if they will have any difficulty getting pregnant once they stop using it. The combined pill contains two synthetic hormones, oestrogen and progestogen; it is taken for 21 days followed by a seven-day pill-free interval which gives a withdrawal bleed (not a true period). The Pill works by inhibiting the secretion of FSH and LH from the pituitary gland so that ovulation stops and by thickening the cervical mucus so sperm cannot swim through easily.

The Pill suppresses ovulation and some women are at their most fertile as they come off it and the ovaries 'kick start' again. Indeed, there are some studies[1] that suggest that the Pill can actually boost fertility, by preventing ovulation and preserving better-quality eggs for use later on.

But for other women, their periods do not resume for many months or years even and it is not possible to predict how any individual's body will react.

Research on the Pill[2] gives us a fuller picture of its effect on fertility. These studies suggest that among previously fertile women who stop taking the Pill in order to conceive, the majority delivered a child within 30 months. Although these statistics seem to bode well, it was found in another study of 'older' childless women, aged between 30 and 35 that they experienced a marked delay when trying to conceive when coming off the Pill. Fifty per cent of these women took a year longer to get pregnant – sometimes taking as long as 72 months – than those of the same age who had not been using the Pill.

Few women, least of all those over 35, want to risk waiting six years once they start trying for a baby. Also, there have been no similar studies on women older than this and logic would suggest that the figures would get worse, not better.

A more serious threat to your fertility is the fact that the Pill may increase your risk of cervical cancer if you take it for more than five years.[3] In addition, fertility threats like diabetes, obesity and uterine fibroids are sometimes aggravated by the Pill.

So should you take the Pill? The choice, of course, is yours, but the chance that you could be one of those women who experience a long delay in conceiving once you come off the Pill would seem to suggest that switching to a more natural form of contraception as part of your pre-conceptual care routine is a good idea. My suggestion, therefore, is to come off the Pill at least three months before you want to conceive and there are two reasons for doing this.

The first is to make sure that your periods start as soon as possible and you know that you are ovulating. If you are not you can then try herbs like agnus castus or dong quai (see pages 87–88) as these can help to get your cycle going again and avoid wasting time.

The other reason for coming off the Pill at least three months before trying to conceive is that it can cause you to become deficient in a number of important nutrients including magnesium, vitamins B1, B2, B6, vitamin E, folic acid (crucial in preventing spina bifida) and zinc (the most important nutrient for fertility).[4] The Pill can also affect blood sugar balance which is significant because nutritional deficiencies and blood sugar imbalances are both threats to your fertility (see pages 14–34).

OTHER METHODS OF CONTRACEPTION

The mini pill

The progestogen-only pill or mini pill has an efficacy rate of 98 per cent, higher in women over 35 but lower in women who weigh over 70kg. It lacks the oestrogen component of the combined pill and works by thickening the cervical mucus so that sperm can't enter the womb. It interferes with the sperm's motion through the fallopian tubes but, unlike the combined pill, does not inhibit ovulation.

The mini pill needs to be taken every day without a pill-free break and must be taken within three hours of its due time to be effective. Possible side effects include menstrual irregularity or total absence of periods and an increased risk of ectopic pregnancy.

Return of fertility The contraceptive effect of the mini pill is short-lived and fertility may return within 12 hours of a missed pill. There is no evidence to suggest any delay in fertility or harmful effects on an unborn baby if taken by mistake in early pregnancy.

Injectable hormones (Depo-Provera)

This contraceptive injection is a slow-release (depot) of a synthetic progesterone (progestogen) every two to three months and has an efficacy rate of 99 per cent. The progestogen released inhibits the release of LH and FSH so the ovaries are not stimulated. One of the most common side effects is absence of periods (amenorrhoea) by the end of the first year of use with some women developing amenorrhoea immediately. Long-term absence of periods is associated with an increased risk of osteoporosis – especially in smokers.

Return of fertility Research[5] shows that women trying to conceive after stopping depot progestogen take at least four months longer to become pregnant compared with those stopping other methods of contraception. In some cases fertility may take up to a year or longer to return so it is not a method I would recommend for women who want to conceive, and in fact would not be a contraception I would recommend in general anyway.

Implants

Progestogen implants are matchstick-size rods that are implanted under the skin of the upper arm. They release progestogen for up to five years, which thickens the cervical mucus and stops ovulation occurring in most women. It has a near perfect efficacy rate with few side effects and is suitable for women who do not want to become pregnant for at least three years.

Return of fertility Once the implants are removed by a doctor, fertility is usually restored in most women within three months. One type of hormonal implant which consists of six small tubes instead of one has recently been discontinued due to health and safety concerns and because users were reporting excessive bleeding.[6]

Female sterilisation
Around 30 per cent of women who feel their family is complete opt for sterilisation. Changes in their personal circumstances, however, result in 10 per cent of these women requesting a reversal. In female sterilisation (tubal ligation) the fallopian tubes are cut, tied or cauterised in a short operation under general anaesthetic. This means that the egg and sperm can't meet. Depending on the method used for the sterilisation the reversal procedure for women under the age of 35 has about a 70–80 per cent success rate. If pregnancy does occur the chances of having an ectopic pregnancy are increased so you need to go for an ultrasound scan as soon as you suspect you are pregnant to make sure that the baby has implanted in the womb.

Return of fertility The procedure should always be considered permanent but tubes can be reunited using microsurgery. Reversal tends to be more successful in women under 35 and success depends very much on the skill of the surgeon and the original operation technique used. One in 300 women becomes fertile again without a reversal, because the tubes can regrow and attach to each other again.

Male sterilisation
Male sterilisation or vasectomy has a near perfect efficacy rate. In this procedure the vas deferens is cut under local anaesthetic. Like female sterilisation the procedure should always be considered permanent.

Return of fertility Reversal is possible but does not guarantee restored fertility. If the reversal is within two years there is a 90 per cent chance of restored fertility and a 50 per cent chance within ten, although sperm production may be poor. About 60 per cent of men develop antibodies to their own sperm afterwards (see page 158) and this can also prevent fertilisation; in order to conceive an ICSI treatment (see page 185) would be needed.

Intrauterine device (IUD)
The intrauterine device, also known as the coil, has an efficacy rate of 99 per cent. Most devices have a flexible plastic frame wound with copper, which can cause a slight inflammatory reaction in the womb, making it unreceptive to a fertilised egg. The coil is inserted into the womb with a recommended life span of three to five years.

Return of fertility The IUD can cause heavy periods so blood levels need to be checked for the possibility of anaemia if you are trying to conceive. Once the IUD is removed fertility usually returns immediately. Pelvic infection can be more likely for women using an IUD, so if you want to use this device it would be better to wait until after you have completed your family. If an IUD is left in place after an accidental pregnancy there is more than a 50 per cent risk that the pregnancy will end in miscarriage. For all these reasons if you have been using a coil and want to start a family my advice would be to have the coil removed at least three months before attempting conception.

Intrauterine system (IUS)

The progestogen-impregnated IUD (coil with reservoir containing the hormone progestogen) has an almost perfect efficacy rate and combines the effects of an IUD with other progestogen contraceptive methods. Cervical mucus is thickened so that it is impenetrable to sperm. It remains effective for up to five years before needing to be replaced. Commonly reported side effects include irregular or absent periods, headaches, breast problems, skin problems, mood swings and nausea.
Return of fertility Usually fertility returns within weeks of removal.

Barrier methods

Barriers methods such as the male and female condom, diaphragm and cervical cap prevent sperm from entering the cervical canal and spermicides kill sperm. When a barrier method is combined with a spermicide they have an efficacy rate of 95–98 per cent as opposed to 85 per cent for spermicides alone. However, incorrect use and the risk of condoms slipping or bursting increase the failure rate to between 11 and 15 per cent.
Return of fertility Fertility returns immediately and research has shown no increased risk to babies born accidentally using barrier methods with spermicides. Using a male condom with spermicide can also reduce the risk of catching STDs. Because they contain no hormones, have no side effects and are easy to use condoms are a good choice for couples who are doing a three- to four-month pre-conception care programme before trying for a baby. Although the success rate is lower than with other contraceptives. With a long-term partner, it is better to use spermicide-free condoms, as the most common spermicide used – nonylphenol – is actually a xenoestrogen (see page 92) and can, therefore, have a hormonal effect on both the man and the woman.

Withdrawal method

This is without doubt one of the oldest methods of contraception. It involves a man withdrawing his penis just before he is about to ejaculate so that sperm does not reach the vagina. If practised carefully the success rate is surprisingly high and if no other form of contraception is available this is certainly better than nothing. However, the risk of premature ejaculation or sperm coming into contact with the vagina is still extremely high so perhaps not the best choice of contraception in the pre-conception period.

Fertility awareness or natural family planning

By learning to recognise your body's fertility signals you can determine when you are going to ovulate and avoid intercourse during this time. If used correctly this method of contraception has a 97 per cent efficacy rate with no impact on fertility. It can even promote fertility by allowing intercourse to be timed on the most fertile days of the menstrual cycle. Obviously user failure depends very much on motivation and the accurate use of this method. Couples who do conceive accidentally using this method are sometimes concerned that intercourse early in a woman's cycle would involve aged sperm and intercourse after ovulation would involve an aged egg but there is no evidence to suggest health risks to the baby.

QUICK GUIDE TO RETURN TO FERTILITY AFTER USING CONTRACEPTION

Modern medicine offers us many choices when it comes to highly effective contraception but if you want to become pregnant in the near future it is wise to consider the amount of time it typically takes to return to normal fertility. Keep in mind, though, that the figures below *are* averages and some women's bodies may take much longer to respond.

~ Oral contraceptives: 1–4 months
~ Depo-Provera: 3–18 months
~ Implants: 1– 4 months
~ IUD: 1 month
~ IUS: 1–4 months
~ Barrier methods: immediate
~ Fertility awareness: immediate.

FERTILITY AWARENESS OR NATURAL FAMILY PLANNING

To become aware of your fertile times when you want to try for a baby and infertile times if you are using fertility awareness as a method of contraception you need to understand the signals your body sends out. Once you have learned to recognise them you can pinpoint the time when you are most fertile and most likely to get pregnant.

Let's first take a look at what happens in a normal female hormonal cycle because this will help you to understand what your body's signals actually mean. (See also the anatomy of the female and male reproductive systems, pages 195–203.)

The menstrual cycle can vary from 21 days to 40 days. Its length is calculated by counting the first day of bleeding as day 1 and then the very last day before the next bleed or period. The average menstrual cycle is commonly described as 28 days, although this may be true for only one in ten women.

Your monthly cycle is governed by the reproductive hormones, the main ones being oestrogen, progesterone, follicle-stimulating hormone (FSH) and luteinising hormone. In a monthly cycle, lasting approximately 28 days, the first half, called the follicular phase, starts on the first day of your period and lasts for about 14 days. At the beginning of each menstrual cycle, oestrogen and progesterone levels are low and FSH is produced by the pituitary gland in the brain which controls the whole endocrine (hormone) system. This triggers ovulation by stimulating the ovaries to produce oestrogen and the lining of the womb starts to thicken as it prepares to receive a fertilised egg. Oestrogen levels continue to rise until the pituitary gland releases LH which triggers ovulation. The egg (ovum) is then released from a follicle in the ovary and passes down the fallopian tube.

After ovulation at around day 10–14, comes the second half of your menstrual cycle called the luteal phase. Here the ovaries produce progesterone which prevents further ovulation from taking place in that cycle. If fertilisation does not occur the lining of the womb breaks down and menstruation takes place about 14 days after ovulation. At the same time there is a dramatic and rapid fall in oestrogen and progesterone and with this drop in hormone levels, the cycle begins all over again. If fertilisation occurs, however, the egg implants itself into the wall of the womb where it begins to develop. Fertilisation takes place in the fallopian tube and once this happens the empty follicle which releases the egg forms the corpus luteum which produces progesterone. This is an important hormone in fertility because it maintains the womb lining during the second half of the cycle in readiness for a fertilised egg. It is also responsible for maintaining pregnancy for the first twelve months until the placenta takes over.

CHECKING YOUR FERTILITY

During your menstrual cycle your hormones bring about many changes in your body from the obvious bleeding during a period to changes in your body temperature. Since the egg only survives for up to 24 hours and the sperm can live for five days in alkaline mucus, there is only a short window of opportunity each month in which you can conceive. Therefore, understanding and recognising the changes in your body when you are ovulating, or about to ovulate is one of the most important ways to pinpoint the best time to have intercourse in order to conceive.

The two main changes that you can learn to observe to monitor your fertility are in your cervical mucus and in your basal body temperature (BBT). Changes in your cervix, breasts and even your mood can also give you clues about your fertility.

Cervical mucus

The mucus-secreting glands which line your cervical canal produce mucus continuously but this fluid undergoes important changes during your menstrual cycle.

During the first half of your cycle your mucus is thick and sticky. It forms a plug over the cervix, which stops sperm entering. It also makes the vagina acid which can kill off sperm quickly. Then about three or four days before ovulation, as your oestrogen levels increase, the mucus becomes clear and stretchy and there is more of it.[7] This fertile mucus turns the vaginal fluids alkaline and provides nourishment for the sperm in the form of increased amounts of sugar, amino acids, salt and water. Surrounded by this mucus sperm can live for up to seven days. Another interesting aspect of the fertile mucus is that it forms swimming lanes or canals through which sperm can pass effortlessly and quickly. It may also act as a filter allowing healthy sperm to travel forward but trapping unhealthy sperm and blocking their passage – there are always some unhealthy or abnormal sperm in semen. Once ovulation takes place, however, progesterone levels increase and the mucus becomes thick and sticky again – protecting the cervix from sperm.

Some women only produce fertile mucus for a few days each month so it is vital to recognise when it is happening. As ovulation approaches your vagina will probably feel more lubricated and wet. The mucus discharged from your vagina increases in quantity and becomes clearer and stretchy. This is fertile mucus.

To identify fertile mucus for yourself, after passing urine blot your vaginal mucus with white toilet paper. Lightly apply a finger to the mucus then pull gently away to test its ability to stretch. If it feels slippery like raw egg white and can stretch between your first finger and thumb up to several inches before it breaks, it is fertile mucus. If it is dry, thick, sticky or crumbly (like glue) and opaque white or yellow in colour it is the more acid, infertile mucus. As it changes to become fertile mucus, this is a sign that ovulation is about to take place.

Bear in mind that there are other factors that may also affect cervical mucus which you need to be aware of. For example, if you have thrush or some other vaginal discharge it won't be so easy to see the changes in your cervical mucus. Also the day after having intercourse you may notice some white or clear discharge – this is liquefied semen which disappears within 24 hours but can easily be confused with cervical mucus. If you are sexually aroused you may also get profuse vaginal lubrication which can be confused with fertile mucus. Try the glass of water test – vaginal secretions on your fingers will dissolve in water but cervical mucus stays in a blob. Tight and synthetic underwear can also make you feel sweaty and damp and tampons and panty liners can also dry your vulva making it hard to detect cervical mucus changes. Finally, hormonal contraceptives and many drugs can affect your cervical mucus, making it difficult to interpret fertility signals. If you are taking any medications in the pre-conception period, always seek advice from your doctor about how they can affect your fertility and mucus.

Anything that can have a 'drying effect' on the body in general could affect cervical mucus, e.g. antihistamines, diuretics, etc. And as we want the vagina to be alkaline around the fertile time of the month, it is better generally to eat a more alkaline diet. A high-protein diet, especially animal protein, will make your body more acid, so aim for a 70–80 per cent alkaline diet (higher intake of fruit and vegetables) and only 20–30 per cent acid. Stress can also make your body more acid, so do what you can to lower your stress levels.

It might help to keep a daily record of your cervical mucus and also to record when you have had intercourse and whether a condom was used as this can affect the discharge the next day. Pelvic-floor exercises (where you tighten the pelvic floor muscles and hold them for a few seconds as if you needed to use the toilet but had to wait and then relax) can also help you to detect changes in your mucus. When mucus is at its most fertile you will notice a slippery feel between your legs as you use these muscles but at other times this area will feel drier. Pelvic-floor exercises can be done anywhere at any time and in any position – while you are queuing at the cashpoint, waiting in traffic or chatting on the phone. Getting good control of your pelvic-floor muscles can also heighten pleasure for you and your partner during intercourse.

Cervix position

Every month your cervix also changes position and you can feel these changes yourself. First, make sure your fingernails are short and clean, empty your bladder and wash your hands. Then place your index finger in your vagina until you feel your cervix. (If you are not sure what you are looking for, see page 196.)

Towards the end of your period your cervix will be lower in your vaginal canal than normal and the opening will be closed. If you try to touch it you will feel as if you are touching the tip of a small nose. Closer to ovulation, however, oestrogen levels rise and the cervix moves higher in the vaginal canal, making it harder to reach. It also begins to soften and open, like parting lips, making it easier for sperm to enter. After ovulation the cervix lowers again and closes; mucus prevents sperm from entering.

Basal body temperature

Normal body temperature averages at about 98.6°F for women, but soon after ovulation it rises between 0.5 and 1 degree and stays that way until menstruation begins (basically the same as incubating an egg). The rise in temperature is due to the hormone progesterone and is a sign that ovulation has taken place. Charting your temperature each day can tell you that you are ovulating and when. For example, on the graph below ovulation occurred around day 18 and it is on the days just before this that you should be at your most fertile. Using this method you should have intercourse every other day from about day 11 to day 18.

Because the temperature reading has to be your basal body temperature it needs to be measured first thing in the morning. Normal body temperature rises as the day goes

TEMPERATURE CHANGE OVER ONE CYCLE

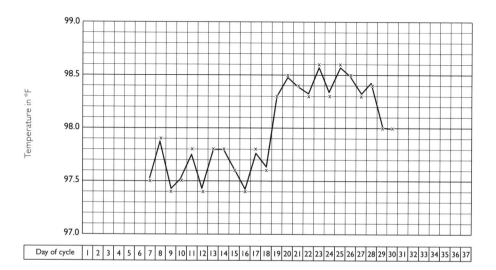

on so you need to take it at the same time each day in order to detect a routine rise as opposed to one that occurs after ovulation.

Take your temperature immediately on waking, before you get up or go to the toilet. If you can, use a Fahrenheit thermometer as the rise in temperature after ovulation is easier to see. If you use a mercury thermometer it must be a special ovulation one with an expanded scale. If you don't want to have to get up and write down your temperature, electrical digital thermometers register your temperature within a minute and have a memory. Plotting your temperature on a graph is the best way to detect changes in your cycle. Don't forget though that many factors can affect your temperature such as alcohol, exercise, stress, anxiety, fever, drugs and shift work so in my opinion detecting changes in your mucus is probably the better method of the two.

Other fertility signs
Some women feel a sharp pain or dull ache on the lower side of their abdomen when they ovulate; it can be a short twinge or last for 24 hours and feel really uncomfortable. A tiny loss of blood may also occur in some women around ovulation but it is always wise to check with your doctor that this is in fact due to ovulation if you get spotting in the middle of the month. Some women also say that their libido increases around ovulation and that their breasts feel tender afterwards. Tender breasts may be due to progesterone circulating in your body after ovulation.

USING FERTILITY AWARENESS TO GET PREGNANT

As you've seen the most important day to have intercourse is when you notice that your cervical mucus is slippery, clear and stretchy. If you examine your cervix as well you will also notice that it softens and opens up during your fertile phase. The rise in your BBT is a reassuring sign that ovulation has occurred although you need to know that this temperature rise sometimes doesn't show up until 24 hours after (which is too late for fertilisation but can help you the next month if your cycle is fairly regular).

To optimise your chances of conceiving you should have intercourse when you notice a wet feeling and slippery mucus. To make the most of fertile mucus you should have intercourse on the first day that you feel wet and notice a stretchy discharge. Then you should try to have intercourse every other day while the mucus stays wet and stretchy. A 48-hour break between intercourse allows time to maximise sperm volume.

Learning to check your cervical mucus is extremely helpful if you have irregular cycles or may miss a period, because the mucus will let you know that ovulation is impending. Hopefully, also by following the recommendations in this book, you will start to have more regular cycles. Cycles can vary from 21 to 40 days and they are classed as regular if your periods occur at roughly the same time each cycle.

Although fertility awareness or the use of ovulation kits (described below) can be incredibly helpful if you want to get pregnant quickly, don't let it take over your life. The last thing you want to do is lose spontaneity or enjoyment in your lovemaking or make your partner feel as if he is nothing more than a breeding stud.

Home testing kits
Ovulation predictor kits help you to predict when you are going to ovulate by measuring the LH surge in an early-morning urine sample. A dipstick will change colour after being dipped in your urine when levels of LH are increasing. When an LH surge is detected it is likely you will ovulate within the next two to three days.

You can buy ovulation kits from most chemists and they come with full instructions and are extremely easy to use. There are usually five dipsticks in a kit and the recommendation is to keep testing until the LH surge is detected. The downside is that they can be expensive and if your periods are irregular, or if you have polycystic ovaries and high LH levels as a result, the results may be misleading and inaccurate. Some patients have also found that if they buy cheaper ovulation kits they end up getting false positives when compared to the more expensive ones.

Persona is an ovulation prediction device that uses samples from your urine to measure LH changes during the month. A dipstick is inserted into the device and if a green light goes on it suggests the possibility of getting pregnant is low. If a red light shows, however, getting pregnant is more likely, and on days when ovulation may be occurring an O will also appear on the display. Although it is marketed as a method of contraception it can be extremely useful if you are trying to get pregnant.

There are also tests which use saliva to pinpoint ovulation. The theory with these is that saliva changes structure with rising levels of oestrogen and this can be seen under a pocket microscope. The dried saliva shows a dotted pattern on non-ovulating days and a clear pattern around ovulation. It is possible to measure oestrogen and other reproductive hormones in saliva and I use these tests regularly in the clinic but I have not had any experience of using saliva for predicting ovulation or any feedback from patients. This is not to say they don't work but it would be interesting to use the saliva tests alongside the urine ovulation kits to see the correlation.

If you want to use ovulation kits to help you get pregnant there is no reason why not. The important thing is to find a way to identify, through mucus testing or using a dipstick test, the days of your cycle on which you are fertile and most likely to get pregnant. Getting the timing right can make the difference between conceiving or not.

OVULATION

Don't worry if you don't seem to ovulate every cycle, this is fairly common. If, however, this is the case for two to three consecutive cycles arrange for a blood test to measure progesterone – the hormone released from the ovary when you have ovulated. By measuring the progesterone level on day 21 (seven days after ovulation when it is at its peak level on a 28-day cycle) you will know whether or not you have ovulated. But not everyone has a 28-day cycle so 'day 21' is not set in stone – if yours is a 35-day cycle where you might be ovulating on day 18, the progesterone test should be on day 25.

If your cycle is irregular the chances are you are not ovulating on a regular basis. A check-up will help to establish if your irregularity is due to some underlying condition such as PCOS or thyroid disorders but if no cause is found fertility-awareness techniques, such as checking your mucus every day, can still help you to recognise when you are most likely to be fertile. Alternatively, you could do a monitored cycle with ultrasound and saliva (see page 146).

THE BEST TIME TO HAVE SEX

Although making love in the week before and at the time of ovulation may well help to increase your chances of conception, a study conducted by the US National Institute of Environmental Health Sciences (NIEH) in North Carolina suggested that fertility-day timing is far less predictable than experts had thought, which will come as a great relief to women with irregular cycles who have no idea when they ovulate. Gynaecologists have always known that ovulation day can vary a little even for women with super-regular cycles, but they never realised how often this happened and to what extent. Now the NIEH study figures suggest that even in healthy women who have no fertility difficulties only one in three ovulates between days 10 and 18 of their menstrual cycle, let alone on day 14. Research by Canadian scientists published in 2003 in the journal *Fertility and Sterility*[8] also suggests that women experience far more hormonal surges each month than previously believed and that each has the potential to produce an egg.

Not surprisingly, this has caused quite a stir among fertility experts. But where does it leave a couple trying to get pregnant? Learning to read your ovulation signals *can* and *does* help, but at the end of the day there may not in fact be an ideal time to have sex. The best advice therefore is probably the oldest: to maximise your chances of pregnancy have as much sex as possible (on alternate days in order to build up sperm), whether your cycles are irregular or regular. Lots of sex will help to normalise your cycles. It will help your partner too, as abstaining stacks up larger volumes of sperm but at the same time reduces its quality and poorer-quality sperm are less likely to make you pregnant, no matter how many of them there are.

Research[9] also shows that women who have regular satisfying sex, with intercourse at least once a week, have more regular menstrual cycles and fewer fertility problems than those who don't. In addition, a satisfying sex life can be a wonderful way to reduce stress and therefore encourage fertility. How? In much the same way as exercise reduces body tension that can interfere with hormone production, so can sex. The tension-releasing power of orgasm can be so great for some people that its effects are more powerful than a tranquilliser.

COMMON FERTILITY MISCONCEPTIONS

When you're trying for a baby you may encounter a surprising number of old wives' tales or theories about the best way to conceive. Your partner may be told to abstain from sex for seven days before or you may be told to put your feet up immediately after intercourse. When you were trying to avoid pregnancy you may also have been given lots of advice, for example that jumping up and down after intercourse can help to prevent pregnancy. But how many of these are true or simply popular misconceptions?

Myth You cannot get pregnant the first time you make love.
Fact You most certainly can get pregnant the first time you make love.

Myth You cannot get pregnant from intercourse during menstruation.
Fact Although it is unusual, it is not impossible to fall pregnant, especially if you have a short cycle, e.g. 21 days.

Myth Jumping up and down after intercourse prevents pregnancy.
Fact Jumping up and down won't make any difference.

Myth You only need to use precautions the first time you make love in a session.
Fact You need to take precautions every time.

Myth Women over the age of 35 cannot get pregnant easily.
Fact Although fertility does decrease with age, as many as one in ten children are now born to women over the age of 35.

Myth The worst contraceptive pills to miss in the pack are those in the middle.
Fact Missing pills at any time in the pack is risky but not taking the first or last is most risky. If a woman is taking the contraceptive pill and misses any pills she should take additional precautions.

Myth A woman needs to have an orgasm to get pregnant.

Fact Although a man usually needs to have an orgasm for conception to happen, it is not necessary for a woman to have one. But it can help if a woman can climax after the man because the contractions of her womb and vagina help to suck the sperm up into her cervix. Without orgasm they will still get there, just not so quickly.

Myth Regular cycles are a sign of fertility.

Fact Women continue to have regular periods well into their 40s, but the quantity and quality of their eggs has already declined and ovulation may not be occurring. It's a misconception that if your cycles are still like clockwork, everything's fine.

Myth It doesn't matter who's on top.

Fact Although technically this is true, according to some experts the positions both you and your partner assume during and right after making love can significantly affect the passage of sperm into your vagina to your fallopian tube. The man-on-top position has the best chance of getting a woman pregnant, but there are no studies to prove this. The rationale is that this position allows for deep penetration so the man's sperm can be ejaculated as close to the cervix as possible. This gives the sperm cells a flying start on their long journey, as the closer they are to the ripe egg waiting in the fallopian tube several centimetres further up in a woman's body, the more likely they are to reach it.

Logically, any position that goes against gravity, such as woman on top or having sex sitting or standing up, discourages the sperm's journey upward and is thought to deter conception. If a man enters a woman from behind, especially if she is kneeling in front of him so she is at an angle with her bottom higher than her head, it is said to encourage conception. Making love in the spoons position (both partners facing the same way with the man penetrating the woman from behind) is not thought to be such an effective baby-making position because the penetration angle is not so deep. The chances might be maximised if the woman leans the upper half of her body a little away from her partner, pushing her bottom against him.

The only exception to this would be if you have a retroverted uterus. Normally the womb is in an up-and-down position or tipped towards the front but in some women, the womb tilts backwards. It does not affect fertility but sometimes can make intercourse painful or difficult. The best positions for intercourse if you have a retroverted uterus are either rear entry or with the woman on top and this will help the sperm to get as close to the cervix as possible.

Myth Your partner should abstain from intercourse for seven days before your most fertile time.

Fact Some research suggests that after seven days' abstinence sperm count and volume are significantly greater than if a man abstained for only three, but more recent research contradicts this suggesting that more than one or two days' abstinence can be detrimental to sperm quality.[10]

Myth Putting your legs up against a wall after intercourse for at least half an hour can increase your chances of conceiving.

Fact Studies[11] show that the best and fittest sperm reach the fallopian tube in five minutes and the rest usually get there within 45 minutes. So as long as you don't leap up or go to the toilet the moment you are finished, you probably don't need to be stuck on the floor or bed with one eye on the clock. In any case, it is the fastest and fittest sperm that you want to fertilise the egg.

Myth Adoption relaxes you, and brings back your fertility.

Fact Many of us have heard stories how a couple spontaneously conceive after adopting a new baby. For many couples, adoption is a very satisfying answer to infertility, but it does not increase subsequent fertility. We don't hear stories about the thousands of infertile couples who do not conceive after adopting, just the interesting few who fortunately do.

Myth If you've already conceived once and had a healthy baby, getting pregnant again will be a cinch.

Fact This is one of the biggest misconceptions my patients have and secondary infertility is a real phenomenon. The fact is, you're older the second time around and your reproductive system changes over the years. A study of about 2,000 couples undergoing in vitro fertilisation (IVF) found that pregnancy attempts were 70 per cent more likely to fail if the man was 40 or older. So if you do plan on having more children, don't wait too long. If you're approaching 35 or older you should consider getting started on baby number two sooner rather than later.

Myth Having had a miscarriage makes it harder to conceive.

Fact Miscarriage, which occurs in 25 per cent of all pregnancies, does not affect a woman's ability to get pregnant. The problem is staying pregnant. You usually need to have had three miscarriages in a row to get investigations started on the NHS, but if you have had just one I would suggest that you put into place the recommendations in Step 1 and take a three-month break while you both get yourself into good health.

Myth Trying too hard can stop you getting pregnant.
Fact If you have been trying to conceive for any length of time you have probably been given advice from well-meaning or not-so-well-meaning friends or family. You've probably heard, 'You need to relax and stop trying so hard' or, 'I know a couple who tried to get pregnant for years but as soon as they decided to adopt, guess what? She got pregnant!' Then, add to that the recent research suggesting that stress significantly impacts on fertility and limits the success of assisted conception. It may make you wonder whether there really is something in it.

Although stress may have an impact, it is more likely that stress is the result of infertility not the cause. Most couples conceive within a year of trying and for those who don't there is often an identifiable physical or nutritional cause. It is also simply not true that fertility improves when you stop trying. The percentage of women getting pregnant after adopting is about 5 per cent, which is the same as women who have infertility and do not adopt.

But what about the theory that having too much sex stops you conceiving? It's another common misconception because the more sex you have when you are trying for a baby the more likely you are to get pregnant. Most experts recommend having sex at least every other day during a woman's fertile period.

To sum up, the difference between a couple that conceives when trying and a couple that does not is not based on how hard they try. Indeed, to suggest that not trying increases your chances of getting pregnant only adds to the frustration of couples trying to conceive. Exactly how do you try less when you desperately want a baby? If you and your partner have been trying to conceive for over a year consult your doctor for fertility treatment options. The bottom line is that there is no such thing as trying too hard for a baby.

step seven
fertility tests

If you've been trying for over a year to get pregnant, or you are over 35 and have been trying for six months, then you should start looking into whether there is a problem and what can be done about it. Your doctor may refer you to a consultant at your local hospital or a specialist fertility clinic for further investigations. Treatment for infertility within the NHS is limited and waiting lists vary. When you see your doctor ask him/her what is available locally on the NHS and if there is a limit to the help you'll receive. Check too about the cost of any prescribed drugs. Will the practice pay or will the bill come to you? If you want treatment privately, your doctor will tell you about clinics in the area. Ask them for information about the tests and treatments they offer, waiting times and the costs involved. Then ask your doctor to refer you to the clinic you've chosen. If you are over 35 don't be fobbed off; be assertive because time is not on your side. If your doctor tells you to come back in six months insist on being tested now.

MOVING ON

When you are referred for fertility investigations, you may feel apprehensive, fearing the unknown, wondering what is wrong with you or your partner. Try to be reassured by the tests, however, because if you find out what is wrong then you can do something about it. And with a diagnosis of unexplained infertility, where there is no medical reason why you are not conceiving, you need to look at the other factors covered in this book, such as nutritional deficiencies and lifestyle which may be stopping you getting pregnant. During the testing keep talking to your partner and if it all seems overwhelming try to keep a sense of perspective. It might seem as if everyone else is getting pregnant but as many as one in six couples have problems conceiving and you just happen to be one of them. If possible, try to limit yourself to one hour a day dealing with and thinking about fertility testing and remember that your relationship is important and you need to keep the lines of communication open at all times because your partner has feelings too. And whatever you do, don't forget about making love as there is always the possibility of achieving a spontaneous pregnancy at any stage on your fertility journey.

FERTILITY TESTING

Fertility tests consist of a progressive series of checks on both you and your partner to eliminate any potential causes of infertility. After each test is complete the results will help to decide what the next stage of testing should be. Although the tests tend to follow a chronological order there will be variations from couple to couple as the nature of fertility problems will be unique to each couple. At all times try to take things one step at a time and be prepared to be assertive if you need to and to ask questions if you feel uncertain. It is so important to have a plan of action so that boxes are ticked off in the order they need to be, giving you the confidence that you are covering everything and also that you are not wasting time. For some couples I have seen in the clinic, it has taken three years to get a diagnosis of unexplained infertility, and that, in my opinion, is not acceptable.

Understanding what each fertility test is for will help you to feel more in control and less fearful of what is happening to you. That's why this step in my fertility-boosting plan focuses on the various tests you and your partner might have to undergo so that you are prepared for every eventuality.

FERTILITY TESTS FOR WOMEN

A number of tests may be necessary and they tend to fall into four distinct groups:

1 Hormone testing, e.g. FSH, LH, oestradiol, progesterone, and tests for ovarian reserve, i.e. AMH, etc. (see page 46)
2 Monitored cycle
3 Tubal and womb investigations to see if disorders or malformations of the reproductive system are preventing conception
4 Immunological testing to check for blood-clotting factors, etc.

Hormone testing
Typically the first step in any fertility screening for a woman is two blood tests to help determine whether there are any hormonal imbalances or disorders that might be preventing pregnancy.
The first blood test is done on day 2 or 3 of your cycle and should check for:
~ FSH
~ LH
~ prolactin
~ oestradiol
~ thyroid function.

If there is a suspicion of PCOS (see page 170) then testing for male hormones (androgens) would normally be added to the screen.

The other blood test is typically done on day 21 of a 28-day cycle, i.e. seven days after ovulation (or later or earlier if your cycle is longer or shorter), and tests for levels of progesterone to see if ovulation has occurred and whether the level is high enough for successful implantation.

FSH (follicle-stimulating hormone) This hormone stimulates the growth and development of the follicles on the ovary during the follicular phase or first half of the menstrual cycle. The test must be done on day 2 or 3 of the cycle, so while you are still having a period (day 1 being the first day of your period). It has been argued that a high FSH level shows not only reduced ovarian reserve (fewer eggs left) but also poor egg quality. It is normally suggested that if the FSH level is over 10iu/l on days 2 to 5 of the cycle you should not have IVF or ICSI treatment as the response to the drugs is going to be poor. I must stress that an FSH level over 10 does not stop you getting pregnant naturally.

MY STORY I started thinking about having children when I was 37 as I'd had a busy and stressful career with a lot of travel. By the time I was 38 my periods seemed a bit irregular but I had not taken much notice. But when I was not pregnant by 39, I went to a fertility clinic for advice. I was told that I was peri-menopausal, had a less than 1 per cent chance of conceiving and that I should really consider egg donation. This news was devastating. My FSH was very high (55), indicating that my ovarian reserve was low and that IVF with my own eggs would not be successful because I would not respond to the drugs.

By the time I was 40 I was having bad night sweats (up to ten a night) and my periods were few and far between. Thinking that this was definitely the menopause, I went to one of Marilyn Glenville's talks on 'Natural Alternatives to HRT'.

I then decided to go to Dr Glenville's clinic for a consultation and was sent a questionnaire which asked about my diet and lifestyle. My husband and I also did a mineral analysis test. We were both put on a programme of supplements to correct the deficiencies shown up on the mineral test. I was also given a combination of organic herbs to help with hormone balance and my hot flushes vanished. We also made changes in our diet by cutting out alcohol, coffee and tea.

My husband also eliminated fizzy drinks and we started to eat more healthily. Three months later and we were still both being monitored at the fertility clinic as we were just about to proceed with egg donation with my sister. My husband was amazed as his sperm count had increased by over 30 per cent. On the morning of my appointment at the fertility clinic my period had not arrived. I just thought it was late again but before I left for the appointment I did a pregnancy test and it was a strong positive. When I got to the clinic, they did a blood test which confirmed the news. I now have a beautiful baby boy.

What does a high FSH level mean? On the first day of your period, FSH (follicle-stimulating hormone) is released from the pituitary gland. Its role is to stimulate a group of follicles to grow on the surface of the ovary. So FSH should be low at the beginning of the cycle because it is only just beginning to rise. If the level is high at this time, it means that the ovaries need more stimulation in order to grow follicles for ovulation. This can be a reflection of ovarian reserve because if there are fewer eggs, the pituitary gland has got to release more FSH in order to stimulate those eggs; in effect the body has to work harder to ovulate. When the IVF drugs are given which, again, are supposed to stimulate eggs to grow, the response is going to be poor.

But there are two things that need to be considered. Firstly, when FSH is measured between days 2 and 5 of the cycle, other hormones are usually also measured then as well, e.g. prolactin, thyroid, oestrogen (oestradiol), LH. If you have an FSH level of below 10 but a high oestrogen level (over 180pmol/l or 80 pg/ml in the USA) this can be a false reading for FSH. The higher oestrogen level will push the FSH level down. If your oestrogen level is high you need to repeat the test earlier in the cycle, so if you had the blood test on day 3 repeat it on day 2 the following month; once the oestrogen level is below 180 you will be seeing a true reading for your FSH.[1]

Secondly, and this is extremely important, a high FSH level may only be reflecting a measure of quantity (how many eggs you have left) rather than quality (how good they are). It does not lead to reduced fertilisation rates or an increased risk of miscarriage. It is true that there will be a lower pregnancy rate because of fewer eggs produced but even women under 38 with an FSH of up to 20 have a 20 per cent chance of giving birth from IVF treatment, which is comparable with the national average.[2]

When you follow the recommendations in this book you will be improving the quality of your eggs, so even if you have fewer left, if the quality is good there will be a much greater chance that they will be fertilised and that you will become pregnant.

LH (Luteinising hormone) LH is released by the pituitary gland to stimulate ovulation. A surge of LH in the middle of your cycle triggers ovulation. This is the hormone that is measured on the urine ovulation sticks. LH is tested on days 1 to 5 and unusually high levels may indicate polycystic ovary syndrome or PCOS (see page 170).

Prolactin This hormone is released by the pituitary gland and in increased amounts when breastfeeding. High levels can stop ovulation and menstruation. One of the symptoms of high prolactin levels is the secretion of breast milk and this can occur even in women who have not recently had a baby.

If high prolactin levels are found, further tests would be organised to rule out any factors that may be causing this overproduction, such as an underactive thyroid (hypothyroidism) or a tumour on the pituitary gland. It is also possible to suffer from high prolactin levels without any medical reason. One of the factors involved in raised levels that cannot be medically diagnosed is stress.

Oestradiol (E2) This hormone causes the womb lining (endometrium) to thicken ready for implantation. It naturally decreases as a woman approaches the menopause so she cannot produce enough oestradiol (one of the forms of oestrogen) to balance FSH which rises. It is typically measured in a blood test on day 1 to 3 of your cycle. Ideally, both FSH and E2 should be fairly low as high levels can indicate diminished ovarian reserve.

Thyroid hormones Thyroid-stimulating hormone (TSH) is produced by the pituitary gland. It is responsible for controlling thyroid function which is important for all metabolic processes in your body. A TSH result that is over the expected range can indicate an underactive thyroid, especially if combined with a below-normal T4 (thyroxine) level. An underactive thyroid (see page 166) is linked to infertility.

Androgens Androgens are male hormones that every woman produces. They are typically tested for at the beginning of your cycle to determine if you have PCOS – a common hormonal imbalance in which large amounts of LH prevent ovulation and cause the ovaries to secrete higher than normal levels of androgens.

Progesterone This works with other hormones to prepare your body for pregnancy and also prevents any further ovulation taking place in that cycle. Progesterone is produced by the empty follicle which becomes the corpus luteum, once the egg is released from the ovary and levels continue to rise for several days. If fertilisation does not occur, progesterone levels drop and you get your period. If levels continue to rise a pregnancy has occurred. A blood test on day 21 (in a 28-day cycle) indicates whether or not ovulation has taken place.

OVULATION TESTING To achieve pregnancy you need to know when and if you are ovulating and the most reliable way to determine this is to undergo a series of diagnostic tests. These tests are usually done in conjunction with noting cervical mucus, using ovulation kits or taking your temperature. (See pages 131–136.)

A transvaginal ultrasound is an important tool for aiding in the diagnosis of PCOS (along with blood tests) and to determine if you are ovulating. This method uses sound waves to produce images of your reproductive organs. A hand-held cylindrical instrument called a transducer is inserted into your vagina to measure your ovaries and check the womb (uterine) lining. The ultrasonagrapher can examine the size of your ovaries to see exactly how many follicles are developing and how big they are. (Optimum follicle size for conception is about 16–22mm in diameter and the womb lining should be about 10–12 mm thick to sustain a pregnancy.)

MONITORED CYCLE

If you have not had any fertility examinations (except for maybe a 'Day 21' blood test for progesterone), this is one of the best first step tests you can take. Monitoring your cycle is an excellent investigative tool and a useful aid to treatment. It means that by the end of one cycle you know your fertility status and, with the help of the clinic, what your plan of action should be. Monitored cycles are organised by my clinics and combine a number of the most important fertility tests all in one cycle:

Day 1 of your cycle: the first day of your normal menstrual flow.

Day 2 to 3 – blood test: this is the follicular-phase blood test (see above).

Day 6 to 8 – first ultrasound scan: this checks the structure and function of your womb, ovaries and pelvis. It also looks for abnormalities such as polyps, fibroids or endometriosis (adenomyosis).
Predicting ovulation – a further two to three scans: these monitor the development of the ovarian follicles as they prepare to release the egg. They look for the ripening of

the womb lining in terms of both thickness and structure and also help to predict the time of ovulation. So while you get an idea of when ovulation is going to occur from the scans, you can also use a predictor kit at home and check your cervical mucus (see page 131). The ultrasound scans are the most accurate way to predict ovulation, but if the predictor kit and/or mucus check are giving you the same information as the scans you can use one or both of them in future months when you are not being scanned to give you a good idea of when ovulation will occur.

Tubal patency: the check for tubal patency HyCoSy (see page 150) can be performed just before ovulation so you get the information on whether your tubes are clear in this one cycle.

After-ovulation scan (approximately seven days after): this scan checks the environment for nurturing a fertilised egg. It looks at the corpus luteum development in the ovary where progesterone is produced. It also checks the ripening of the womb lining ready for implantation.

Monitored cycle saliva testing for hormones: at the same time as you are doing the monitored cycle with ultrasound scanning, you would perform a test which maps your hormones over the entire cycle. Blood tests, e.g. 'Day 21' are just a snapshot of the hormones measured on that particular day of the month, but it is also extremely useful to see what the pattern and the relationship of your hormones are like over one complete cycle. Because this is inconvenient and uncomfortable to do with blood testing (you would need to have blood taken at least eleven times in one month), the hormones oestrogen, progesterone and testosterone are measured in saliva and eleven samples are collected over the cycle at specific times and then posted to the lab. The results of the saliva testing are then looked at in relation to the ultrasound-monitored cycle. (See Home testing kits, page 135 for more details.)

It is interesting to note that 46 per cent of women under the age of 40 whose pelvic scan is normal (i.e. no womb abnormalities, etc.) conceive within three months of having the monitored cycle.

Making sense of the results
Should your blood tests and/or ultrasound scan suggest that you are not ovulating due to hormonal imbalance, you will be recommended the most suitable treatment options to adjust that imbalance. Often changes in diet and lifestyle are enough, so keep

FEMALE HORMONE PROFILE

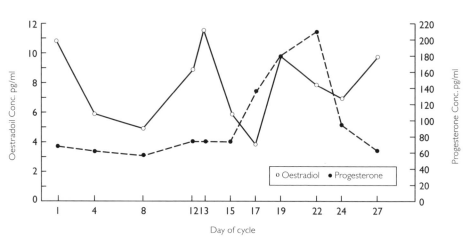

Sample cycle mapping levels of hormones using saliva

following my advice in Steps 1 to 5. You may also be referred for assisted conception, such as ovulation stimulation (see Step 8, pages 176–194).

If your FSH levels are too high there is a possibility that your ovarian reserve is low. You would not be advised to try IVF because with a high FSH, over 10, you may not respond well enough to the fertility drugs. But age is also a factor here. Young women with high FSH levels produce fewer eggs so it does affect their response to the drugs and IVF cycles can be cancelled, the same as with older women (over 35). However, with younger women if eggs can be retrieved and embryos transferred back then the success of the IVF and the pregnancy rates are the same as in young women with normal FSH levels.[3]

Many clinics will not allow women to undergo IVF or ICSI cycles if their FSH is over 10, making this a cut-off point. But the reason for this could be concern that this will affect the clinics' overall success rate.[4] By only selecting women with a low FSH certain clinics are skewing the statistics so that they come out higher on the league tables than others who may be treating a broader selection of women.

If prolactin levels are raised you should be referred to an endocrinologist who will check for any problems with the pituitary gland and who may recommend medication. You should also be referred to an endocrinologist if the thyroid tests are abnormal.

If androgens are too high more tests will be carried out, such as blood (glucose) sugar and insulin tests, to see if you have PCOS (see page 170).

If progesterone levels are too low the blood test will be repeated at another point in your cycle and then, if they are still low, you will be referred to a fertility specialist. A result that is higher than 30 nmol/l suggests that ovulation is occurring but a value of around 50 or more is preferable for implantation to occur.

POST-COITAL TEST This test used to be very popular and was used to assess the cervical mucus and the nurturing and mobility of sperm through the mucus. The couple performs sex around ovulation and then the woman goes to the clinic within 12 hours, where a sample of mucus is taken and examined under a microscope. The test checks whether, if the man produced a good sperm sample, radical changes have taken place in it following contact with the cervical mucus.

Few clinics still do this test for a couple of reasons. Firstly, the timing has to be so precise that not many clinics, especially NHS, can organise it. Secondly, research does not show that it changes pregnancy rate, so it is not cost effective. The *British Medical Journal* concluded that 'routine use of the post-coital test in infertility investigations leads to more tests and treatments but has no significant effect on the pregnancy rate'.[5]

ULTRASOUND SCANS The ultrasound scan is used to check if follicles, which should contain eggs, are being produced and whether you are ovulating. It is also useful for looking at ovarian reserve because during the first half of the cycle the scan can examine the size of the ovaries and the number of measurable small (antral) follicles (developing eggs).

Tubal and womb (uterine) investigations

After your hormone levels have been assessed the next phase in your fertility testing is to look for any structural (anatomical) problems that may be preventing implantation and for blockages in your fallopian tubes that could be stopping the egg or sperm progressing. Blocked fallopian tubes are said to account for 20 per cent of female infertility and can be caused by congenital abnormalities, infection, pelvic inflammatory disease and scar tissue from previous surgery. The following tests will normally take place in the first part of your menstrual cycle, to ensure that you are not already pregnant.

Hysterosalpingogram (HSG) This is a routine test where a dye is passed through the fallopian tubes to check they are not blocked or malformed. A small tube is inserted into the cervix through which liquid dye is squirted. X-rays are taken as the dye passes through to see if there are any obstructions, scar tissue or uterine abnormalities such as fibroids or polyps (small harmless growths). The procedure is painless but you may feel uncomfortable and cramping can occur. Some studies[6] suggest that the likelihood of pregnancy following this procedure increases – probably because it helps to remove minor blockages. If a blockage is found a laparoscopy (see below) will be recommended to find out more; if no blockage is found a laparoscopy may still be advised to check the womb.

HyCoSy (Hystero-contrast Sonography) This is similar to the HSG but has the advantage of using a trans-vaginal ultrasound instead of x-rays to assess the tubes. A very fine solution of air bubbles is injected through the cervix into the womb. The solution will be seen to flow through the fallopian tubes if they are patent (open).

Laparoscopy Performed under general anaesthetic, a laparoscopy uses a thin telescopic instrument to view the reproductive organs through a small cut below the navel. It checks for scar tissue, endometriosis, fibroids or any abnormality in the shape or position of the womb, ovaries or fallopian tubes.

Hysteroscopy A viewing instrument called a hysteroscope (a lighted scope) is inserted via the cervix into the womb to check for irregularities or scar tissue.

Immunological testing
If you have a history of miscarriage or fertility problems that have yet to be identified you may be sent for an immunological screening. This will involve two blood tests, carried out six weeks apart. As you'll see on page 167, certain immune reactions may result in your body rejecting a fertilised embryo. Numerous studies[7] have found abnormal levels of certain antibodies in women with repeated IVF failure or miscarriage.

If the testing reveals that you have high levels of antiphospholipid or anticardiolipin antibodies you will be given a low-dose aspirin every day to thin the blood. Heparin may also be offered. Antibodies cause your blood to thicken and this increases the chances of miscarriage dramatically as it reduces blood flow through the placenta and increases the risk of clots. Antibodies may also trigger inflammation in the womb which can put the foetus at risk and if any inflammation is detected you may be offered steroids to reduce this. Also levels of natural killer cells may be checked for. For more information, see page 168.

YOUR DIAGNOSIS

If all this testing yields a diagnosis this may bring with it a sense of relief because it means you can have a treatment action plan to maximise your chances of conception. Whether you are diagnosed with endometriosis or a hormonal imbalance such as PCOS that inhibits your fertility, it is important that you are told what this means and how it impact on your fertility. You need to understand all the implications so that you set about finding the best way to improve your diet, health and lifestyle to help you get pregnant as quickly as possible.

At my clinics we help you through the maze of testing, investigations and diagnosis and work out an individualised plan of action that means you get to see the relevant specialist quickly and that no time is wasted (see page 224).

If you are not given a definite diagnosis this can be bewildering and it is more important than ever for you to pay attention to your diet, lifestyle and stress levels, as the positive changes in Steps 1 to 4 of my fertility-boosting plan could well make all the difference. Approximately 30 per cent of patients who have been trying for a baby for a year or more and have been unsuccessful are diagnosed with unexplained infertility, so please don't feel that you are alone.

CAUSES OF MALE INFERTILITY

Although traditionally considered a woman's responsibility, female factors are the cause of 35–40 per cent of fertility problems, male factors are the cause of 30–35 per cent of cases and in the rest the problem is a combination of the two. So it's crucial that men have fertility testing as well as women and also that they do it as early as possible because many conditions affecting male fertility are symptomless, requiring skilled investigation to identify them.

There are many theories about the causes of male infertility but unfortunately in at least 30 per cent of cases the cause is not determined. The remaining 70 per cent are believed to be caused by abnormal sperm, hormonal imbalance, varicocele, infections, sperm obstruction, damage to the testes, autoimmune problems and other physiological issues – such as ejaculation problems and genetic problems.

ABNORMAL SPERM

It typically takes at least three months for sperm cells to mature, ready to be ejaculated and that's why it is vital for your partner to put healthy diet and lifestyle changes into place at least three months before trying to conceive. In order to impregnate a woman, a man must produce sperm that is capable of reaching the egg and fertilising it. For this to happen sperm must be sufficient in terms of both quantity and quality; if it is abnormal or unhealthy in any way this can affect a couple's fertility.

One thing that has become evident is that more and more men are coming to me with fertility problems which simply confirms what research is already indicating – that sperm counts are falling.[8] Some experts believe that there is a strong link between declining sperm counts and environmental toxins.[9] Some toxins cause free radical damage and can be responsible for larger numbers of abnormal sperm and even DNA damage within sperm. (Free radicals are controlled by antioxidants which is why I always urge men with abnormal sperm readings to take an antioxidant supplement to give them the chance of producing more normal sperm.)

CASE STUDY A couple came to see me who had been trying to conceive for three years. After numerous medical investigations it was discovered that the husband had a very low sperm count of 1.5 million (should be at least 20 million to conceive) with 95 per cent of these being abnormal. The motility of his sperm was also low at only 27 per cent. They were told that they had no hope of conceiving naturally and that they should go for IVF.

Because of the man's poor semen analysis they had to have an ICSI cycle. Fourteen eggs fertilised and two were put back into the woman's womb without success. The ICSI was draining both physically and emotionally and the couple were devastated by the outcome. Apart from the stress and the invasive nature of the procedure it had cost them more than £3,000.

When they contacted me, following all this, I recommended they perform a hair mineral analysis ahead of their first consultation to detect whether there were any deficiencies that could be impacting on their ability to conceive. They were delighted at how simple and non-invasive the test was after all the blood tests, injections, prodding and poking they'd endured over the previous three years.

Two weeks later they met with the clinic's nutritionist who spent a full hour with them going through their medical and fertility history and their plans and goals. One of the first areas she addressed was helping the woman to eliminate the toxins in her body from the drugs used in the IVF treatment.

The hair mineral analysis showed that the woman was low in the minerals zinc and magnesium and her husband was low in zinc, selenium and magnesium. The nutritionist explained how important zinc was for both of them, particularly for the man in whom it was needed to enable the head of the sperm to penetrate and fertilise the egg.

The nutritionist referred the husband to a microbiologist who performed an infection screen which came back positive. He was then referred on to a urologist who prescribed antibiotics to clear the infection. Immediately this reduced the percentage of abnormal sperm, but motility and count were still low.

Having followed an eating plan to maximise their fertility and taken nutritional supplements tailored to their needs, they were asked to come back for a follow-up appointment and to arrange another semen analysis before this so they could see what had happened in this time. This analysis showed that the percentage of abnormal sperm had dropped to 90 per cent, the count had increased to 6 million and motility to 35 per cent.

Six months on she was pregnant! The clinic recommended an early scan at five weeks to reassure them, then at 12 weeks they had another consultation to review their progress. The hair mineral analysis was repeated so the nutritionist could make the necessary adjustments and talk them through the final two trimesters and the birth of their baby boy.

HORMONAL IMBALANCE

In about 5 per cent of cases the cause for a poor semen analysis is hormonal. Hormone imbalances can affect a man's fertility in much the same way as they affect women. FSH and LH are released from the pituitary gland (as in women) to stimulate testosterone production and a lack of these hormones can result in poor sperm production – a condition known as hypogonadotropic hypogonadism. General hormone imbalances that affect sperm production in a negative way can also be caused by conditions such as liver disease, thyroid disease and diabetes. Age also has an impact on hormonal imbalance in men as do obesity, chronic stress and intense physical exercise. Once again we come back to the idea of balancing hormones so that they can function efficiently and do the job they are meant to do. This can be achieved by aiming for optimum health through changes in diet and lifestyle, so that the body has tools to balance itself.

VARICOCELE

This condition is similar to varicose veins but involves enlarged veins around the testes which can inhibit sperm production and perhaps motility. There is some evidence that a varicocele can overheat the testes, causing problems with fertility; however, many men have completely harmless varicoceles that have not affected their fertility. Unfortunately doctors cannot predict which men with varicoceles will benefit from having them treated, but if you are having trouble conceiving, it is probably wise to do so. This normally involves tying off the affected veins.

DAMAGE TO THE TESTES

Men with damage to the testes or who have testicular failure will produce poor-quality or no sperm because the release of the hormones they produce is affected. Testicular failure may be due to genetic or birth defects, sexually transmitted infections or mumps, if it occurs before puberty. Also, any condition such as influenza which causes a fever or temperature of more than 38.5°C may damage sperm production for three to four months. Physical trauma such as violent kicks to the groin can damage the testes.

EJACULATION PROBLEMS

Retrograde ejaculation is a condition in which the semen is pushed back into the bladder at the point of ejaculation because the muscles that pump the semen through the penis don't work properly. Retrograde ejaculation can be caused by conditions that damage nerves such as diabetes. Fortunately, it is possible to recover sperm from urine and use it in assisted conception techniques such as IUI.

Blockages in the male reproductive system, frequently caused by STDs can also cause problems with ejaculation and in some cases surgery is the answer. Some men also have no vas deferens, the tube connecting the testes to the penis (see page 201), so that sperm cannot travel down to be ejaculated. Impotence or inability to get an erection and ejaculate may be caused by medical conditions such as diabetes, but they can also be caused by stress and anxiety, which could be helped with counselling.

FERTILITY TESTS FOR MEN

So as you can see, just as for women, there are a number of factors that can cause or contribute to fertility problems in men and your clinic should eliminate as many as possible to determine the cause. Testing for men will typically involve a semen analysis; then if there are any problems with the sperm further testing is usually carried out and can involve: hormone testing, a physical examination, scanning, biopsy and genetic tests.

Though some men may want to put off being tested out of embarrassment, early testing can spare their partner a great deal of unnecessary discomfort, distress and expense. For example, studies show that there is an increased risk of miscarriage if there are sperm abnormalities.[10] This is why it is absolutely crucial for both partners to be in optimum health before conception and, if you are having problems conceiving, why *both* of you need to go for fertility testing.

SEMEN ANALYSIS

The first thing your partner needs to do is to have a semen analysis. This is best done in a specialist clinic as the quality of the results can vary considerably. If your partner feels uneasy, remind him that a semen analysis is a commonplace test, and the results could save months of worry and stress.

If the first semen analysis is not good, the man is often asked to repeat the test.

A semen analysis assesses the sperm for quality and quantity. This simple non-invasive procedure involves the man masturbating into a sterile container. Ideally the sample should be collected at the lab where the analysis will be done because it can deteriorate if it has to be transported from home (both temperature and time can affect it). The man needs to abstain from sex ideally for two to three days (not less than two and not more than five, otherwise sperm motility is affected). For men who feel uncomfortable producing a sample by masturbation or for whom religious beliefs prohibit this, special condoms can be provided by the clinic to collect the sperm. It is important that ordinary condoms are not used as spermicides and lubricants on the condom will affect the sperm and can give a false reading.

The lab will analyse the sample, looking at the following factors:
~ sperm count (the number of sperm per millilitre – should be over 20 million per ml)
~ sperm motility (the percentage of sperm moving – should be more than 50 per cent)
~ sperm morphology (the percentage of abnormal sperm – more than 15 per cent should be normally shaped)
~ seminal volume (should be between 2 and 5ml)
~ pH (should be between 7.2 and 8.0)
~ white blood cells (should be fewer than 1 million per ml)
~ round cells (should be fewer than 5 million per ml)
~ agglutination (sperm clumping – there should not be any)
~ antisperm antibodies (if less than 50 per cent may not affect fertility)
~ debris (graded 0–4, 0–1 being normal)
~ liquefaction (sample should be liquid within 60 minutes)
~ viscosity (the 'thickness' of the sample – should just say 'normal').

SEMEN ANALYSIS

Duration of abstinence (days) 3   Interval between ejaculation and start of analysis (min) 60

SEMEN ANALYSIS	PATIENT VALUES	REFERENCE (WHO 1999)
Macroscopic examination		
volume (ml)	2.48	$\geq$ 2mls
appearance	normal	Normal
liquefaction	complete	Complete
viscosity	normal	Normal
pH	8.0	7.2 – 8.0
debris	not significant	
agglutination	none seen	
Motility (% spermatozoa)		
(a) rapid progression	23	
(b) slow progression	16	
(c) non-progressive	31	
(d) immotile	30	
Vitality (% live)	78	> 50%
Antisperm antibodies (% bound)		< 50% may not affect fertility
MAR test for IgA	< 1	$\geq$ 10%
MAR test for IgG	< 1	$\geq$ 10%
Concentration (x 10^6/ml)		
count/ml	30	$\geq 20 \times 10^6$/ml
total count in ejaculate	74.4	$\geq 40 \times 10^6$/ml
Other cells (x 10^6/ml)		
round cells	1.6	<5 $\times 10^6$/m
polymorphonuclear leucocytes	< 0.01	<1 $\times 10^6$/ml
Morphology (%)		Multicentre studies in progress
normal	2	$\geq$ 15%
abnormal	98	
head defects	98	
midpiece defects	41	
tail defects	26	
cytoplasmic droplets	2	
teratozoospermia index (TZI)	1.70	1.6 or less

Comment: High abnormal frms, mostly tapered, pyriform heads. Fructose test was positive.

What do these factors mean?

Sperm count This is measured as how many sperm there are in 1 millilitre of the ejaculate. Ideally it should be over 20 million, but if a woman is fertile it is still possible for her to conceive with a man whose sperm count is right at the bottom end of normal, i.e. 20 million, as long as the sperm are healthy.

Sperm motility With the motility, 50 per cent must have progressive motility with at least 25 per cent having rapid progression – it makes no difference if a man has a high sperm count if the sperm can't swim to reach the egg. I have seen results where more than 50 per cent have been immotile.

Sperm morphology This factor looks at the shape of the sperm where more than 15 per cent should be normal in shape (oval head, normal mid-piece and long tail). That does not seem a lot when you think then that means 85 per cent of them are abnormal. Higher numbers of abnormal sperm can lower the fertilisation rate and affect motility.

The percentage of normal sperm can be classified in two ways. The World Health Organisation classification can grade sperm on the borderline of normal as being normal. But a stricter classification called the Kruger strict criteria for assessing sperm morphology includes a detailed morphological interpretation and gives an in-depth description of the shape of the sperm (see sample semen analysis). Under the Kruger strict criteria, a borderline sperm would be classed as abnormal. The Kruger criteria say that if the percentage of normally shaped sperm is lower than 14 per cent fertilisation would be unlikely. Using the Kruger criteria has been helpful in predicting the ability of the sperm to fertilise the egg.

Abnormal sperm can have malformations in the tail where it can be coiled, thickened, stumped or even have a double tail and the sperm can't move. This is more common in older men. Also, instead of the head being oval, there can be a round head, pin head, large or even double head and this will not be able to fertilise the egg. There are suggestions that the level of abnormal sperm is more important than the count, because nature's survival of the fittest rule will kick in, so if the sperm are not normal, fertilisation may be prevented or a miscarriage may occur. Many poor morphology problems are due to lifestyle factors, excess exercise, heat and too much oxidation, so the recommendations in the first part of this book can make a real difference to producing normal sperm.

Seminal volume This is the amount of ejaculate in a sample. If the volume is too low this can interfere with the transportation of sperm and they may not reach the cervix. It can also indicate infection, retrograde ejaculation or an obstruction in the epididymis. If the volume is too high this can dilute the density of the sperm and affect their motion.

pH The pH of the semen should be alkaline because of the seminal vesicle secretion and this alkalinity protects the sperm from the acidity of the vaginal fluid. If the pH is too acidic there could be a problem with the function of the seminal vesicle.

White blood cells and round cells If either of these is high, this could indicate an infection as the body is mounting an immune system attack.

Agglutination This means that the sperm are clumping together, which can prevent forward motion and stop the sperm swimming up through the cervix. Agglutination can indicate that there is an immunological problem and that the man's body is producing antibodies to his own sperm.

Antisperm antibodies Antisperm antibodies can cause agglutination or even prevent fertilisation because they stop the sperm being able to penetrate through the cervical mucus. They can occur after a vasectomy reversal where sperm has 'escaped' into the bloodstream and the body views it as a 'foreign object'. Sperm antibodies can also be produced after an infection. The MAR (mixed antiglobulin reaction) test for sperm antisperm antibodies is usually done as part of the semen analysis. If the MAR test is less than 50 per cent it may not affect fertility.

The recommended treatment is usually steroids but they have side effects such as weight gain, stomach bleeding and depression. It is also thought that steroids will only work if the antisperm antibodies are found in the blood and not just in the sperm. Normally an ICSI treatment would be recommended if sperm antibodies are found.

Debris If significant debris is seen this can indicate an infection or inflammation of the prostate (minor amounts of debris is common and normal). The man is then asked to ejaculate more frequently to see if that clears the debris and then repeat the test to see if it has made a difference. If not further checks on the prostate are recommended.

Liquefaction The normal criterion is that semen should be liquid within 60 minutes which allows the sperm to swim efficiently. If liquefaction is incomplete (within 60 minutes) this may hinder sperm motility.

Viscosity If the viscosity is high then this may stop the sperm from moving efficiently. It could also indicate a problem in the prostate.

MEDICAL TERMS USED WITH SEMEN ANALYSIS ARE

Azoospermia No sperm are produced, or the sperm are not appearing in the semen.
Oligiospermia Few sperm are produced.
Astenozoospermia Problems with sperm motility.
Teratozoospermia High levels of abnormal sperm.

While these conditions may be the direct reason that you and your partner can't conceive, they themselves may be caused by an underlying medical condition. The clinic may want to investigate further with blood and urine tests or other procedures.

Also, it would be worth considering a sperm DNA fragmentation test (see page 47) if any of the following applies to you:
~ years of unexplained infertility
~ history of recurrent miscarriages
~ a number of failed IVF or ICSI attempts
~ embryos stop developing during IVF or ICSI
~ the man is over the age of 35.

Although a semen analysis is extremely useful, it does not provide any information about the genetic quality of the sperm. There will always be a certain amount of DNA fragmentation in sperm that is repaired by the egg after fertilisation. Beyond this, however, the repair process does not happen and an embryo may not develop.

The DNA fragmentation test is performed on a sperm sample, collected in the same way as for the semen analysis. With the lab I use, the sperm DNA fragmentation test is performed on the same sample used for the semen analysis and can even be requested a couple of weeks later if the DNA test seems warranted. (See page 224 for my clinic details if you would like this test).

OTHER TESTS
A simple blood test can indicate levels of FSH, LH and testosterone. As we've seen, FSH and LH are important for the development of healthy sperm in the testes and testosterone is also essential.

As with women, if FSH levels are high this could indicate a problem. In men, it indicates that there could be a problem with sperm production in the testes. Testing inhibin B for men is useful where no sperm are found in the semen (azoospermia). If the inhibin B level is greater than 80pg/mL (a normal level for men is classed as 300pg/mL) then irrespective of FSH and testosterone levels, there is a good chance that viable sperm can be removed by a testicular biopsy to be used in an ICSI treatment.[11]

And what is also useful to know is that if men are thinking of having a vasectomy reversal, measuring inhibin B levels first can give an idea of whether it is worth having the reversal done. Inhibin B levels of below 80 are predictive of poor fertility and in that situation it may be better for that man to go for percutaneous epididymal sperm aspiration (PESA) (see page 187) and then have an ICSI cycle instead of going for the vasectomy reversal.

Your clinic may also want to determine whether or not there has been any damage to your partner's testes or any sign of infection. Testicular inflammation can lead to reduced testosterone production and reduced fertility. An ultrasound scan is used to examine the scrotum, testes, epididymis, prostate and seminal vesicles. This can detect infection, inflammation, the absence of vas deferens, obstructions and tumour.

If your partner has a very low sperm count or an absence of sperm due to a blockage the cause could be a chromosome abnormality. Potential genetic problems, such as Young's syndrome, are investigated by means of a blood test. Depending on the results he will be offered genetic counselling and as a couple you should discuss the possibility of an assisted reproductive technique.

CONDITIONS THAT CAN AFFECT FEMALE REPRODUCTIVE FUNCTION

In couples who have been trying for their first baby for over a year ovulatory failure (including PCOS) cause approximately 20 per cent of infertility problems; tubal damage accounts for 15 per cent; endometriosis 5 per cent; and male problems 26 per cent. Approximately 30 per cent is 'unexplained'.

Listed below are the most common conditions that diminish fertility, some of which are directly related to your reproductive organs and some of which are not. Whatever problem or condition you are diagnosed with, always remember the importance of Steps 1 to 4 (i.e. good nutrition, regular exercise and stress management) in your fertility-boosting plan.

Note: if you are diagnosed with pelvic inflammatory disease (PID) or a genito-urinary problem, such as candida, chlamydia, herpes, bacterial vaginosis or gonorrhoea, refer to Step 6.

ANAEMIA

Studies show that anaemia is a common occurrence in women diagnosed with infertility and malabsorption problems like coeliac disease.[12] Iron deficiency is the most common cause of anaemia and other types of anaemia include pernicious anaemia. A woman is diagnosed with iron-deficiency anaemia when blood tests reveal too few red blood cells to carry energising oxygen around the body; symptoms include fatigue, heavy periods, tearfulness and pale skin.

If tests suggest that you are iron-deficient, take extra iron (as amino acid chelate or citrate, not ferrous or iron sulphate as it is less easily absorbed) at 14mg per day. Vitamin C is essential for the body to absorb iron, so for maximum absorption take 1000mg (1 gram) of vitamin C with your iron supplement *on an empty stomach*. Take iron and vitamin C supplements at a different time of day from any others you may be taking as the iron can block their absorption (the same applies to the nutrients in your food).

Try not to drink Indian or regular black tea with your meals, which blocks the uptake of iron from your food. Similarly, phosphates, found in soft fizzy drinks, will prevent iron absorption. Herb teas and fruit juices are fine. Iron-rich foods include green leafy vegetables, parsley, sunflower seeds, dried fruits, eggs, fish, seaweed and nuts.

COELIAC DISEASE

Studies[13] show that coeliac disease – a medical condition caused by an intolerance to gluten which prevents food from being digested and absorbed properly – can cause fertility problems. Symptoms include bloating, unpleasant-smelling stools, anaemia and tiredness. Many nutritional deficiencies have been noted in women with coeliac disease, including folic acid, vitamins A, D and E, zinc and selenium and it is known that many women with this condition have problems getting pregnant. This is yet another indication of the important role nutrients play in increasing fertility.[14]

The disorder is diagnosed by having a biopsy in which a sample of the small intestine is removed for examination. Alternatively a blood test can reveal antibodies to tissue transglutaminase – a highly sensitive marker for identifying coeliac disease (see page 218 for more information about this blood test).

If you test positive for coeliac disease you will have to remove gluten from your diet and you will probably be given dietary advice with your diagnosis. You may also be advised to have a nutritional assessment to ascertain which supplements are required to correct any deficiencies.

DIABETES

Although there is no direct link between Type 2 diabetes and infertility, insulin resistance may contribute to an absence of ovulation and women with full-blown diabetes are more likely to be overweight and to miscarry.[15]

Symptoms include fatigue, blurred vision, excessive urination and constant thirst. A check for sugar in your blood or urine can determine a diagnosis. Mild cases of diabetes or insulin resistance can be treated with dietary measures but more severe cases will need medication to control blood sugar levels.

ENDOMETRIOSIS

Endometriosis is a common but often painful disorder in which cells that usually form your womb lining (endometrium) migrate outside your womb and attach themselves to other organs – most commonly your fallopian tubes, ovaries or the tissue lining your pelvis. When your monthly cycle triggers a period, the migrated womb-lining tissue continues to act in its normal way – it thickens, breaks down and bleeds each month as your hormone levels rise and fall. But because it can't exit through your vagina it becomes trapped and can form scar tissue and even cysts that bind internal organs together and cause pain and fertility problems.

Symptoms include acute pain or cramp in the pelvis (it is believed to be the cause of 80 per cent of pelvic pain), heavy bleeding, severe PMS, mood swings and fatigue. The cause is not known but it is thought to be due to excess oestrogen as well as a weakened immune system, as a result of stress and poor diet.

Good nutrition is considered vitally important in treating endometriosis and the fertility-boosting hormone-regulating diet and supplement guidelines in Steps 1 and 3 will all help to balance oestrogen levels and reduce inflammation.

Supplementing with essential fatty acids may be particularly beneficial. Our bodies produce beneficial prostaglandins from essential fatty acids and these can reduce period pain and have an anti-inflammatory effect. In one study on endometriosis, women were asked to eliminate caffeine, to control blood sugar and supplement with essential fatty acids. The researchers found that with these simple measures the women experienced a significant decrease in their symptoms.[16]

Medical treatments involve painkillers and synthetic hormones to limit the production of oestrogen, but the condition responds well to self-help in the form of a healthy diet, regular exercise and stress management, as recommended in this book.

Fibroids Fibroids (also called myomas) are non-cancerous growths in or on the muscular wall of the womb (the myometrium). Fibroids are given different names depending on where and how they grow. If fibroids protrude into the womb (called submucosal fibroids), they increase the risk of infertility and miscarriage because they may make it difficult for the implanted embryo to develop properly.

Fibroids larger than about 4–5cm in diameter may cause problems during pregnancy as they can prevent the foetus from developing properly by pushing against blood vessels. Fibroids larger than 6cm growing outside the uterus may also block the passage of the egg in the fallopian tube. However, women with small fibroids can have a problem-free pregnancy.[17]

Fibroids are the most common structural abnormality of the uterus and it thought that up to 50 per cent of women between the ages of 35 and 50 may have them. What causes them is unknown but a high-fat, low-fibre diet, weight gain and a female relative with the condition are believed to be contributory factors.

Symptoms include heavy or irregular bleeding, abdominal pain, a feeling of fullness or pressure on the lower abdomen, constipation, the need to pass water frequently, especially during the night when the fibroids exert pressure on the abdomen and bladder infections or irritation.

Polyps are similar to fibroids in that they are benign masses of tissue that grow out of the endometrium and because they cause low-grade inflammation in the endometrium they can act like an IUD in preventing implantation.

Fibroids and polyps are diagnosed via an ultrasound scan and there are various methods of treatment depending on how serious the problem is. If the fibroids are small and not causing any problems then you may simply be urged to improve your diet and take more exercise. Fibroids are oestrogen sensitive so a diet that is high in saturated fat and dairy foods and low in fibre will make things worse because more oestrogen will be circulating in your system.

Changing to a diet rich in whole grains, nuts, seeds, fruit and vegetables, together with oily fish for at least three months will reduce the pain and bleeding associated with this condition. Eliminating refined sugars, dairy products, wheat, chocolate, caffeine and salt, red meat, poultry and alcohol is also advised. Regular aerobic exercise, stress management techniques like yoga and avoiding use of tampons (which may hamper the free flow of blood from the body) are recommended.

Fibroids and polyps can also be surgically removed.

HORMONAL IMBALANCES

A number of hormonal imbalances can play a part in reduced fertility. Their causes vary – they can be due to an underlying medical disorder such as PCOS (see page 170) but they are also closely linked to nutritional deficiencies, an unhealthy lifestyle and high levels of stress and/or toxins. A good diet, regular exercise, supplementation, stress management and a gentle lifestyle detox as recommended in this book are therefore highly recommended if you suffer from any of the following conditions.

Amenorrhoea

This is the medical term for periods that have been absent for more than three months. The absence is not due to pregnancy or menopause but to lack of ovulation and a temporary failure of the pituitary gland. The condition is often a symptom of PCOS or an underactive thyroid but you may also suffer if you are underweight, have just come off the Pill, have extreme emotional stress, are obese, do intense physical exercise or have nutritional deficiencies. Missing the odd period is common but if more than three months have passed since your last one it is important to see your doctor as soon as possible as in rare cases amenorrhoea can also be a sign of serious illness.

If investigations are all clear then the best way to treat this problem is with good nutrition, along with stress management and easing up on exercise and weight loss if you have been overdoing it. Following Steps 1 to 4 of my fertility-boosting plan can help to kick-start ovulation and improve the condition. A good multivitamin and mineral, like the Fertility Plus for women and supplementing with essential fatty acids (like fish oil) is particularly important.

Dysmenorrhoea

This is the medical term for intense pain during menstruation that is felt in the abdomen, lower back and thighs. It is thought to be related to oestrogen and progesterone imbalance and may be associated with endometriosis or pelvic disease. Your doctor may offer you anti-inflammatory drugs or the contraceptive pill which you probably want to avoid if you are reading this book. Once again diet and lifestyle changes are the best way to tackle this condition along with stress management. See Steps 1 to 4.

Luteal phase defect

If the second half of your menstrual cycle after ovulation is shorter than 12 days, it is likely that you are not producing enough progesterone and/or for long enough to maintain a fertilised egg if it implants in the womb. The medical term for this is a luteal phase defect. Progesterone deficiency is thought to be caused by poor secretion of LH by the pituitary gland. Drug treatments may involve progesterone supplementation (as pessaries) during the second half of your cycle. Many clinics do not offer this but I have seen women in my clinics who would not have conceived or stayed pregnant without the use of progesterone support. It is only given when the woman's body is not producing enough of her own, so is basically replacing what is needed in the second half of the month.

Progesterone is a drug given in the UK on prescription and should only be used in a medical setting with monitoring. The pessaries are administered vaginally, so the progesterone goes exactly where it is needed, and it is all done under medical supervision. I would not recommend using progesterone creams that can be bought on the Internet as you have no way of knowing how much is being absorbed through the skin.

Menorrhagia

This is the medical term used for menstrual bleeding which is very heavy. Your periods may be regular but in menorrhagia the flow is excessive and long lasting and may contain clots. Like other menstrual irregularities it is caused by an oestrogen and progesterone imbalance and can lead to anaemia and chronic fatigue in some cases. It may be linked to endometriosis, thyroid problems, fibroids and pelvic inflammatory disease. The diet and lifestyle advice in Steps 1 to 4 of my fertility-boosting plan can help to alleviate the condition.

Premenstrual syndrome (PMS)

PMS has not been directly linked to any fertility problems but in my opinion you should think of it as a wake-up call or warning of possible hormonal imbalances that might be a threat to your fertility. PMS is thought to affect at least one in four women of reproductive age and it is more common in women aged between 35 and 45. It includes a wide range of symptoms, such as cravings, fatigue, mood swings, bloating, breast tenderness, insomnia, irritability, tearfulness, social withdrawal and forgetfulness that occur in the 10 to 14 days before a period starts.

Women whose diet is high in sugar, refined foods, dairy products and animal fat and low in whole grains, fruit and vegetables and who are, therefore, more likely to have low levels of magnesium, zinc, selenium and B vitamins B, C and E are thought to have a greater risk of PMS. As are women who are overweight, sedentary or who suffer chronic stress.

Antidepressants can be used to treat the symptoms but these do not tackle the underlying causes. Good nutrition (in particular eating little and often so that blood sugar levels do not fall too long), along with regular exercise and stress management are effective natural therapies which can help to correct any imbalance.

High FSH levels

FSH levels can fluctuate, especially if you are under a lot of stress, but the closer you get to the menopause the higher they are likely to be. There aren't any symptoms of raised FSH and you may not find out that you have a raised level until a blood test reveals this to you. There also isn't any conventional treatment for raised FSH but the diet and lifestyle measures in Steps 1 to 4 of my fertility-boosting plan may either encourage the level to lower or give you the best change of conceiving naturally (a high FSH does not exclude a natural conception). The average age of the menopause is 51 (when you finally stop ovulating and having periods) but it can happen to a third of all women before they hit 45. Menopause before the age of 40, which happens to about 1 per cent of all women is called premature menopause.

Raised or high prolactin levels

High prolactin levels can be caused by chronic stress, excessive amounts of exercise, anorexia, an underactive thyroid, PCOS, pituitary gland disorders and certain drugs, including antidepressants and blood pressure medication. Loss of libido, menstrual irregularities and in some cases the production of unwanted breast milk are commonly reported symptoms. Conventional treatment will involve drugs such as bromocriptine or cabergoline to bring prolactin levels down. If a tumour in the pituitary gland is the cause it can often be successfully treated with drugs rather than surgery.

Hypothyroidism

Studies show that a shortage of thyroid hormone, a condition known as hypothyroidism, is a contributory factor in female infertility.[18] Symptoms of an underactive thyroid include weakness, memory loss, hair loss, sensitivity to cold, mood swings, weight loss or gain, heavy or irregular periods. It is typically diagnosed with a simple blood test. If you are found to have an underactive thyroid conventional treatment with a daily dose of synthetic thyroxine is recommended. Dietary measures, regular gentle exercise and other positive lifestyle changes as in Steps 1 to 5 of my fertility-boosting plan will also form part of your treatment. It is also important to make sure you get enough of the following nutrients which are all essential for energy production: vitamins B1, B2, B3, B5 and B6, co-enzyme Q10, magnesium, chromium, selenium, zinc and calcium. If you are borderline underactive thyroid, i.e. your TSH level is high but your T4 (thyroxine) level is normal, it is worth seeing a practitioner who could help to turn this around before it becomes a medical problem (see Clinic Contact Details, page 224).

IMMUNE SYSTEM PROBLEMS

Immune problems may account for a large number of cases of unexplained infertility and pregnancy loss. There is a huge amount of information (and controversy) out there on these problems so if you have been diagnosed with one by a blood test to assess your immune system status it is more important than ever for you to seek a second or even a third expert opinion.

Problems with the immune system occur when your body's normal immune response to a pregnancy goes wrong. Your body naturally produces antibodies to fight off infection or foreign substances but during pregnancy your body should respond differently to an embryo and should form a protective blanket around it. Because half the baby's DNA is not yours (it belongs to your partner or sperm donor), your immune system has, in effect, to quieten down in order to stay pregnant and not reject the baby. In some women, however, instead of protecting the embryo their immune system attacks it as if it were an infection or invading organism.

Antiphospholipid antibodies

Antiphospholipid antibodies (APAs) are the most common kind of abnormal immune system problem. Up to 15 per cent of women with a history of recurrent miscarriage have this syndrome – and a 90 per cent miscarriage rate, without treatment. And APAs can also prevent implantation, preventing pregnancy in the first place. Phospholipids are a sort of glue needed in early pregnancy. Some women, however, produce APA blood-clotting antibodies which attack cells that build the placenta and increase the risk of miscarriage.

Anticoagulants help to prevent clotting caused by APA and both low-dose aspirin and heparin (a blood thinner) are often prescribed. Supplements of omega 3 essential fats, vitamins C and E and garlic also help to thin the blood so you should not take these if you are on blood thinners.

Antinuclear antibodies (ANAs)

Antinuclear antibodies are directed against structures within the cell nucleus and can attack the fertilised egg and the cells in the womb. This can prevent implantation and increase the risk of miscarriage. Antinuclear antibodies are often treated with steroids, e.g. prednisone, to suppress the inflammatory process.

Blocking antibodies (e.g. DQ Alpha)

Some women may fail to produce blocking antibodies to stop the immune system from attacking and rejecting the foetus. The problem is when the woman shares the same antibodies with her partner; in other words the couple's DNA is too similar. Normally, the father's DNA in the embryo tells the mother's body to set up a protective reaction around the baby. But when this blocking effect does not happen, the baby is rejected.

The treatment for this is lymphocyte immune therapy in which the male partner or donor's blood is injected into the woman. Common reactions to this treatment include swelling, irritation, and itching at the injection site. Some women run a fever after this treatment.

Natural killer cells (NK cells)

Natural killer cells are important. They make up 50 per cent of all white blood cells and are needed to control rapidly dividing cells like cancer. The theory is that some women produce too many natural killer cells which will aggressively attack any cells that grow and divide, offering protection against cancer but making pregnancy impossible. The difficulty is that often blood samples are taken to measure NK cells but this peripheral blood, as it is called, does not reflect what the NK cells are doing in the womb, as womb (uterine) NK cells are different from those circulating in the bloodstream.[19]

Treatment possibilities for high NK cells are lymphocyte immune therapy, intravenous immunoglobulins, steroids or rheumatoid arthritis drugs. These are powerful drugs but there is actually a natural solution.

Research has shown that fish oil, specifically EPA, decreases NK killer cell activity by 48 per cent. It was interesting to note that the other oils tested – linseed, GLA (e.g. evening primrose oil) and DHA – did not cause any change in NK activity.[20] The dose of EPA used was 720mg; the omega 3 supplement I use in the clinic contains 700mg in just two capsules (Omega 3 Plus).

Research has also shown vitamin E to be beneficial in dampening an overactive immune function.

Th1/Th2 cytokine ratio

The immune system is balanced between two responses, Th1 (autoimmune response) and Th2 (suppressive response). The two should be in equal balance for health and it is thought a dominance of the Th1 response can increase the risk of miscarriage and infertility.[21]

It has also been found that recurrent implantation failure with IVF has been associated with a predominantly Th1 response.[22]

The treatment for this is an anti-TNF-alpha drug or IVIg may also be used. Research into fish oil has also shown that it can inhibit TNF alpha by as much as 74 per cent.[23] It was found that cytokine production decreased as cellular EPA increased.

Thyroid antibodies

Some women produce antibodies that attack the thyroid gland. It has been suggested that these may reflect an abnormal reaction to T cells (a type of white blood cell and part of the immune system) and may be responsible for implantation problems in fertility, recurrent miscarriages and repeated failed IVF attempts.

It has therefore been suggested that thyroid hormone treatment would be beneficial for women producing these antibodies, even when their thyroid hormone levels are normal. But a report by the Royal College of Obstetricians and Gynaecologists showed that the evidence is not there to support the case[24] and that women with thyroid antibodies going for IVF treatment have the same pregnancy rates as women without.[25]

From the nutritional point of view we know that selenium is absolutely vital for the healthy functioning of the thyroid gland. Research has shown that just 200mcg of selenium a day for three months lowered antibody concentrations significantly in people with thyroid autoimmune problems.[26]

The nutritional approach to immune system problems

As already mentioned, treatment for immune system problems is a controversial area and research is still ongoing. You need to talk everything through and work very closely with your doctor and/or fertility specialist and maybe even get a second opinion where needed. Also, be aware that none of these treatments is licensed for use in reproductive medicine and they are very expensive. As with any drug, there are side effects, not only for the woman but for the baby as well. (The effects on the baby are as yet unknown.) My concern is that by effectively suppressing the immune system of the mother, what effect could this have on the baby's long-term health?

The side effects of steroids are well known and the FDA has classified prednisone as a type C drug. This means that its effect on an unborn baby is not known. Adequate human reproduction studies have not been done with corticosteroids and the use of these drugs in pregnancy.

My recommendation for an immune problem connected with fertility would be to look at it from a different angle. Instead of suppressing the immune system, whether with steroids or anti-inflammatory drugs (e.g. those for rheumatoid arthritis), my aim would be to try and regulate the immune function in a more natural way, especially given the unpleasant side effects of many drug treatments.

One of the most interesting pieces of research in this area has focused on vitamin D. Vitamin D is actually not a vitamin. To be classed as a vitamin, a nutrient has to have an essential compound that the body cannot manufacture and so has to acquire from food. Vitamin D functions more like a hormone; the body manufactures it to serve a particular function. While we do get some vitamin D from our diet, the most important source is the amount we produce in our skin following exposure to sunlight.

Vitamin D is known as an immune modulator in that it helps to balance the immune system. There has been a great deal of research on the effects of vitamin D on the prevention of cancer, especially breast cancer. Deficiencies in vitamin D have been implicated in the cause of many autoimmune diseases such as multiple sclerosis, rheumatoid arthritis, insulin-dependent diabetes mellitus, and inflammatory bowel disease[27] and vitamin D regulates the T helper cells and decreases the Th1 driven autoimmune response. Research has also found that vitamin D helps to promote the suppressor Th2 cells that help the body maintain a pregnancy.[28] By effectively making mice deficient in vitamin D they can actually make them infertile.[29]

So before you go down the route of experimental drugs for suppressing your immune function get your vitamin D levels checked. If you are deficient try supplementing vitamin D for eight weeks and then do a re-test. (See page 218 for information on help with testing.)

When selecting a supplement containing vitamin D, choose one where the form of vitamin D is D3 – cholecalciferol. (D2 – ergocalciferol – is not as efficient in helping to correct low levels or deficiencies of vitamin D in the body.)[30]

The other thing I would suggest doing if you have concerns around immune problems is a test for intestinal permeability or leaky gut syndrome (see page 37). It is thought that increased gut permeability may trigger the start of autoimmune problems.

One consequence of a 'leaky gut' is the formation of antibodies which can end up attacking your own tissue. Different people have weaknesses in different parts of the body, so the problem may be centred on the thyroid, skin, joints, reproductive system and so on. With nutritional help it is possible to heal the gut's permeability and lessen the symptoms. (A test for leaky gut intestinal permeability can be organised by post. See page 218.)

PCOS

PCOS (polycystic ovary syndrome) is a common cause of fertility problems. It is estimated that 20 per cent of women have a tendency towards PCOS, while 10 per cent have the full-blown syndrome.

In PCOS the ovaries are much larger than normal and there are a number of undeveloped follicles that appear in clumps. A woman can have polycystic ovaries without having PCOS but all women with PCOS will have polycystic ovaries. These are not particularly troublesome and in many cases will not even affect fertility. The problem starts, however, when the cysts cause hormonal imbalances such as high levels of LH and androgens and blood sugar imbalances or insulin resistance. These problems put together make it difficult for ovulation to occur.

Symptoms vary in severity from one woman to the next and include: irregular or absent periods, fertility problems or recurrent miscarriage, weight gain, facial hair caused by the overproduction of male hormones, oily skin or acne, hair loss and insulin resistance.

Women who smoke, are overweight, have diabetes or a close female relative with the condition are most at risk. It is diagnosed by an ultrasound scan and blood tests. Since the cause is not known conventional treatments aim to reduce the symptoms of PCOS by reducing the masculinising effects of the androgens with anti-androgen hormones, improving fertility problems by inducing ovulation with fertility drugs, resolving the insulin imbalance with insulin-sensitising medication such as metformin and maintaining a pseudo cycle with the contraceptive pill (which is often in combination with the anti-androgen).

Weight loss is strongly advised as studies show this is very effective in treating women with PCOS and infertility.[31] One reason is that weight loss lowers insulin levels, which then reduces the ovaries' production of testosterone. Unfortunately, however, weight loss can be problematic for women with PCOS since weight gain is a symptom of the condition; you need good nutritional help with this as it is a metabolic problem.

NATURAL TREATMENTS FOR PCOS, FIBROIDS, ENDOMETRIOSIS, PMS AND MENSTRUAL DYSFUNCTION Although PCOS, fibroids, endometriosis and menstrual irregularities are classified as separate conditions above they are often triggered by the same mechanism – hormonal imbalance, poor diet, blood sugar imbalances and stress. By getting these back on track it is possible to alleviate or eliminate the problems.

PCOS, fibroids and endometriosis are all linked to oestrogen; fibroids and endometriosis being sensitive to it and PCOS being characterised by high levels of it. When you are overweight you have high levels of circulating oestrogen because it is produced by fat cells, so with all these problems it is important to address the issue of any weight you need to lose. For all these conditions you also need to make sure that your liver is in peak condition. Your liver is your body's waste-disposal unit, not only for toxins and waste but also for hormones. If your liver is not functioning well you may get an accumulation of 'old' hormones left over from each menstrual cycle. The liver deactivates these old hormones and makes them harmless but in order to carry out this conversion your liver needs to get B vitamins and other nutrients from a healthy diet.

By following the fertility-boosting guidelines for blood sugar and hormone balancing through diet in Step 1, exercise in Step 2, supplementing in Step 3 and lifestyle in Step 4, you will positively affect the underlying cause of hormonal imbalances like PCOS.

For example, as far as your diet is concerned, reducing your intake of saturated fat will help to reduce oestrogen. A diet high in saturated fat found in red meat is known to stimulate oestrogen overproduction so a diet free of animal products can help.[32] Saturated fats also produce hormones called prostaglandins which are highly inflammatory and can worsen period pain and endometriosis-related cramps. Increasing your fibre intake will also help to reduce oestrogen levels because the fibre contained in grains and vegetables prevents oestrogens that are excreted in the bile from being reabsorbed back into the blood. Reducing or eliminating sugar and refined foods makes sense because sugar that isn't used as energy gets converted to fat, which then increases oestrogen production.

Alcohol should be avoided because it can compromise the efficient functioning of the liver so that is it less able to metabolise hormones. Also, alcohol (along with caffeine) acts like a diuretic and depletes the body of important fertility-boosting nutrients like zinc.

As with diet, exercise can directly affect oestrogen control according to recent studies.[33] In fact, regular exercise seems to modify a woman's hormonal activity in a beneficial way. Extremes of exercise can suppress ovulation but regular, moderate exercise as recommended in Step 2 can not only help to balance hormones and ease stress but it can also boost mood and overall health and well-being.

Herbal supplements, in particular agnus castus (see page 87) and milk thistle and dandelion which are excellent herbs for the liver can also have a tremendous impact on these conditions and if the problem is long standing it would be worth seeing a qualified practitioner for a personal consultation.

RECURRENT MISCARRIAGE

A miscarriage is the loss of pregnancy before the first 24 weeks of pregnancy. (A loss after that is called a stillbirth.) Approximately half of all eggs that are fertilised never make it to a viable pregnancy. In these cases most women never know that they are pregnant or that the heavy period they just had was a very early miscarriage. It is estimated that one in four women will lose a baby in the first trimester and about 1 in 200 couples will have more than two consecutive miscarriages.

Women considered most at risk of miscarriage include those who:
~ are over 35
~ smoke
~ are very thin or anorexic
~ drink
~ are very overweight
~ are exposed to x-rays
~ spend long periods in planes
~ are exposed to toxins through their daily work
~ have serious illness
~ suffer from genetic disease or blood-clotting disorders
~ use street drugs
~ overuse laxatives that can stimulate the womb
~ have increased levels of homocysteine
~ eat food contaminated with pollutants.

Note: some of the above factors in a woman's partner may also increase the risk.

Fortunately, advances in medicine mean that in 80 per cent of women the cause of miscarriage can be determined and the problem overcome.

Although it is the woman who miscarries it is important that her partner is also investigated and puts in place all the advice and suggestions in the previous sections because a miscarriage will also occur if the sperm is not as good as it could be.

The most common cause of miscarriage or repeated implantation failure is chromosomal abnormality of that pregnancy (not an inherited genetic problem) and the miscarriage is simply your body's way of rejecting a foetus that is not viable (nature's survival of the fittest). Congenital abnormalities of the womb cavity or scar tissue from surgery or infection are also responsible for one in every hundred miscarriages and luteal phase defects, where progesterone levels are too low, are responsible for one in five. Other factors linked to recurrent miscarriage include diabetes, underactive thyroid, infections, blood-clotting disorders (such as antiphospholid syndrome also known as Hughes syndrome) and abnormal sperm or eggs. In 20 per cent of cases the cause is unknown.

CASE STUDY Susan came to my clinic after four miscarriages, with three in the space of just over 18 months. Each had happened at around the same time – six to eight weeks – but with the last one the baby's heartbeat had stopped at around eight weeks and testing on the baby showed up a chromosome abnormality. Both she and her partner were tested for genetic problems and were given the all clear. In between miscarriages she had also an IVF treatment that was unsuccessful.

All the usual miscarriage tests for blood-clotting factors and immune testing were normal. Susan's Day 21 progesterone was good at 60, so a luteal phase defect was not the cause. Her partner's sperm analysis was also completely normal.

By the time Susan came to me for her first consultation, she had found out she was six weeks pregnant and was concerned, given her history. She had been following a sensible diet but had only started taking fertility supplements a week earlier. A mineral analysis test showed that she was deficient in both selenium and zinc. Both of these minerals are powerful antioxidants and are crucial where there is a history of a previous miscarriage especially one with a chromosome abnormality. Both these minerals were supplemented on top of the fertility multivitamin and mineral, along with vitamins C and E and fish oil.

Susan went on to have a beautiful baby boy and wrote to me after the birth saying, 'He is our dream come true and although ultimately it was mine and my husband's success, we honestly believe we wouldn't have got here without you and thank so you much!'

Scientists believe a number of factors may play a part in miscarriages and numerous potential theories and treatments have been suggested, but few are proven by controlled research studies. Some doctors will treat some factors 'just in case', while others await solid proof that treatments work before intervening.

THE MTHFR GENE The MTHFR gene is one of those things that some clinics investigate for and some do not. Methylenetetrahydrofolate reductase (MTHFR for short!) is an important enzyme in folic acid (folate) and homocysteine metabolism. Of course, folic acid is crucial before and during pregnancy as it reduces the risk of neural tube defects like spina bifida in the baby, while higher levels of homocysteine can increase the risk of a miscarriage (see page 00). I would suggest that you ask for this gene to be tested if you have had recurrent miscarriages and all investigations have come back normal, or if you have had a previous pregnancy with a problem like spina bifida or ancephaly.

For many of the women who come to my clinic the problem is not getting pregnant, but staying pregnant. All too often they have been told to keep on trying but new immunology studies[34] show that if a miscarriage is the result of an autoimmune problem trying again and having another miscarriage can just make things worse. So if you have had one miscarriage already, especially if you are over the age of 35, I strongly advise you to have further investigations.

There are a number of treatments available for recurrent miscarriage but certain forms remain controversial. If you have had a miscarriage it is absolutely vital that you seek advice from a specialist clinic and explore all your treatment options carefully. If the problem is a structural problem with the womb this can often be corrected surgically. If the problem is linked to luteal phase defects, progesterone may be prescribed in the first 12 weeks of pregnancy to help maintain the womb lining which sustains the foetus until the placenta takes over.

Don't forget that, as we saw in Step 1, certain nutritional deficiencies and lifestyle choices can increase the risk of miscarriage so it is essential that you follow my fertility-boosting advice in Steps 1 to 4. For example, be sure to include plenty of magnesium in your diet or take supplements as low levels of magnesium are thought to be a factor. Selenium is also important. This protects cell membranes and women with low levels tend to miscarry more often than those whose levels are normal. Research also indicates that women with low levels of co-enzyme Q10 and folic acid (which can reduce homocysteine levels) have an increased risk. Deficiencies in vitamins A, B6, B12, E and beta-carotene have also been linked to miscarriage (see Step 3).

IN CONCLUSION

If tests on you and your partner show a definite reason why you are not conceiving you should be referred for further investigations or, if necessary, assisted conception (see Step 8).

step eight
assisted
conception

The aim of this book is to help you get pregnant naturally and quickly. Some couples will need additional help though, whether due to an inherent medical problem such as blocked fallopian tubes or no sperm found in the ejaculate. In such cases assisted conception is needed. Regardless of how you are going to conceive you should still put into place the dietary, lifestyle and supplements recommendations from Steps 1 to 4. This is important not just to increase the success rate of any fertility treatments but also to give you the best possible chance of having a healthy baby.

It has been found that couples with fertility problems are three times more likely to have a child affected by disorders that include autism, cerebral palsy, mental retardation, cancer and more moderate health problems such as attention deficit disorder, hearing and sight disabilities. The meeting at the American Society for Reproductive Medicine in 2006 was told that the extra risk is mostly caused by health problems that make it hard for couples to get pregnant in the first place. The study is one of the few that has tracked children up to the age of six years from couples who had difficulty conceiving.

TAKING CARE OF YOURSELF

It is easier said than done but whatever treatment you are going through, try to keep stress levels under control. Research shows that those women who are anxious about undergoing in-vitro fertilisation (IVF) produce 20 per cent fewer eggs and have 19 per cent fewer fertilised than those who are less stressed.[1] The stress management tips on page 65 can all help to keep you calm and centred during fertility treatments as can stress-reducing complementary therapies such as acupuncture and massage (see page 72).

THE CLINICS

If you are having treatment on the NHS your options will be more limited but over the last few years a number of private clinics have successfully bid for NHS contracts, so do check this out. Of course, if you go through the private system you will have more choice. When choosing a clinic try to find out about their success rates. Although there are many clinics to choose from they are not all created equal. Some are linked to hospitals while others are private hospitals. Ring up and ask for brochures.

QUESTIONS TO ASK WHEN DECIDING ON A CLINIC

~ Are the consultants specialists in reproductive medicine?
~ What treatment and tests do they offer?
~ Do they have any age restrictions?
~ Do they have a waiting list?
~ Are there any 'hidden' costs? (You need to know *all* the costs as they can mount up very quickly.)
~ Do they offer a 24-hour, seven-days-a-week service so you can be seen right away if need be?
~ Will you be closely monitored when taking fertility drugs?
~ Are the drugs tailored to your own individual response or do they give everybody the same protocol of drugs regardless of age or response?
~ If you have already had one unsuccessful IVF, do they take into account your response on the first one?
~ Is counselling available should you want it and is it included in the cost?

You should try to meet the specialist who would be in charge of your treatment before making a final choice. Ask yourself if you feel comfortable with them. Do they inspire you with confidence? What does your partner think?

The clinic of your choice should give you quality of service (good facilities and clinical, scientific, nursing and administrative staff), convenience (short waiting list, good location and flexible opening times) and value for money (including medication, tests, scans, etc.).

Take your time when you are choosing a clinic. Do all your research, find out about the doctors who would be treating you and ask to speak to former patients. This is a huge decision and it's vital that you feel comfortable with it, so do shop around – you are the customer and you are paying for a service.

BEWARE OF CLINICS' 'SUCCESS RATES' Although clinics are supposed to report accurate success rates this may not always be the case. Remember that IVF is big business; in the UK the fertility industry thrives at £500 million a year and at $2 billion in the USA.

Statistics can be manipulated. Some clinics exclude couples who they think will not have a good chance of success. Or if the problem is too complex, they do not take them on, which raises their success rates. Couples who seem like good candidates for intra-uterine insemination (IUI) may be pushed into IVF (IVF can cost five times more than IUI) which artificially boosts their IVF success rates.

If an IVF/ICSI cycle does not look like it is going well, one of three things could happen:
~ It could be cancelled.
~ It could be 'changed' into an IUI cycle. This means it does not go down as a failed IVF; IUI success and failure do not have to reported because an embryo is not created outside the body so it does not come under the HFEA regulations.
~ It can be classed as a 'trial of stimulation' – just to see how you respond to the drugs – so again it is not a failed IVF.

So when you are considering a clinic, look at their cancellation rates; if they are low compared to other clinics be wary.

Once you've made a choice, if at any time during your fertility treatment you don't feel cared for or listened to be sure to tell someone, such as another doctor, about your concerns. If you are not currently undergoing treatment you can change clinic. Above all, never undergo a treatment if you don't fully understand the possible side effects or the advice you are given. It is the job of your fertility specialist to give you all the information, time and space you need to make one of the most important decisions of your life.

Some couples can feel under pressure to have one treatment after another, especially if they are 'older'. However, given the strength of the drugs used and the emotional rollercoaster that can go hand in hand with fertility treatment, it is better to have a three-month break between treatments. During this time you should carefully follow Steps 1 to 4 of my fertility-boosting plan, allowing your body to get back to normal before being bombarded with drugs again.

DRUGS FOR INDUCING OVULATION

If you are not ovulating but your fallopian tubes and your partner's sperm are normal, the first line of treatment is typically fertility drugs to stimulate ovulation and ensure the release of an egg. Most of the drugs used to induce ovulation have unpleasant side effects, ranging from nausea to mood swings and insomnia, so make sure you ask your specialist to keep you fully informed. Bear in mind, too, that some studies[2] indicate that fertility medication to induce ovulation may be associated with ovarian cancer and ovarian hyperstimulation syndrome – a rare but serious condition in which the ovaries enlarge as a result of fertility treatment and can cause damage to other organs. Bear in mind too that these drugs do not make you more fertile; they only work during the month in which they are taken.

Many questions remain unanswered about the use and side effects of fertility drugs, so my advice is to proceed with caution. For all the promise that reproductive medicine can bring it also breaks many hearts and bears risks that are as yet unknown.

CLOMIPHENE CITRATE

Clomiphene citrate is used to stimulate ovulation if you are not ovulating. Clomiphene is an anti-oestrogen drug that tricks the brain into thinking there is no oestrogen in the blood. Because the oestrogen is blocked, the pituitary gland gets the message to increase the supply of follicle-stimulating hormone (FSH). This then reaches the ovaries and egg production is stimulated. When the clomiphene is suddenly stopped (it is only taken between days 2 and 5 of your cycle) the brain recognises that there is a massive amount of oestrogen and this results in a luteinising hormone (LH) surge that releases the egg from the ovary.

In women who are not ovulating clomiphene citrate results in ovulation for approximately 80 per cent of women, with 40–50 per cent going on to have a live birth.[3] There are several potential side effects including headaches, depression, fatigue and a 5–10 per cent risk of twins or triplets, as clomiphene increases the number of pre-ovulatory follicles and therefore the chance of multiple pregnancy. More serious side effects include ovarian enlargement or hyperstimulation. If there are any changes in your vision or severe headaches when taking this drug, tell your doctor immediately. Clomiphene can also have a negative impact on fertility by causing your cervical mucus to become hostile to sperm and unfortunately it also increases the miscarriage rate.

It can take a few cycles to determine the right dosage for you and because of the potential side effects, the lowest dose of clomiphene that results in ovulation should be used. The usual starting dose is 50mg (one tablet). Success is usually achieved at doses over 150mg (three tablets a day), but the 'more is better' rule does not apply because higher doses can prevent rather than promote pregnancy. The dose needs to be adjusted according to body weight, with heavier patients needing more. Clomiphene should not be taken for more than six months at a time.

If your doctor continues to recommend it after six cycles, it might be wise to seek another opinion. Studies[4] also show that there is an increased risk of ovarian cancer with twelve or more cycles of clomiphene.

Other studies[5] have also shown that when taken with an insulin sensitiser, like metformin, clomiphene significantly increases the chances of ovulation and pregnancy. In addition, some research[6] suggests that using oestrogen supplementation with clomiphene helps to improve the lining of the womb which, in turn, increases implantation and pregnancy rates. Some specialists also use progesterone support to try and offset the higher miscarriage rate with clomiphene.

HUMAN CHORIONIC GONADOTROPHIN (hCG)

hCG is the hormone that makes an ovary release its dominant follicle (the one that is ripest) and also helps to keep your womb lining in place if you get pregnant. The drug hCG is typically used with other fertility medications including clomiphene, FSH and hMG to promote ovulation by triggering an LH surge. Side effects can include multiple pregnancies and ovarian hyperstimulation syndrome (OHSS).

FSH

FSH controls ovulation, in partnership with LH. Because women with PCOS often have an elevated LH level, pure FSH is sometimes given to balance out the LH to FSH ratio. Once there are adequate levels of oestrogen and the follicle develops, an hCG shot is often given to help release the egg. FSH is given by daily injection. Side effects can include mood swings.

HUMAN MENOPAUSAL GONADOTROPHIN (hMG)

This drug is derived from the urine of menopausal women and contains LH and FSH which stimulates ovulation. It is often given for women with absent periods and who have had no success with clomiphene. It is given by injection, usually in the thigh or buttocks. Side effects can be mood swings and there is an increased risk of ovarian hyperstimulation, if not monitored properly, along with multiple pregnancies.

BROMOCRIPTINE

This drug is used if a woman secretes too much prolactin from the pituitary gland. Prolactin is the same hormone that stimulates breast milk and can stop ovulation because it inhibits the release of FSH and LH. This drug is given in tablet form and can cause nausea, headaches, dizziness, fainting and decreased blood pressure.

GONADOTROPHIN-RELEASING HORMONE (GnRH)

GnRH stimulates the release of FSH and LH from the pituitary gland. When women lose large amounts of weight rapidly, or if they have anorexia, the secretion of GnRH decreases and ovulation stops. Because GnRH is released naturally by the hypothalamus in the brain in small amounts every 90 minutes the woman has to wear an automatic pump which releases the GnRH into the skin. It has been found that some men and women with a lack of GnRH lose their sense of smell. This same symptom can also indicate a deficiency of zinc – the most important mineral for both male and female fertility. Side effects include headaches and nausea and there is a tiny risk of multiple pregnancies.

GONADOTROPHIN-RELEASING HORMONE (GnRH) ANALOGUES

These synthetic hormones work in the same way as GnRH. They can be given as an injection or as a nasal spray. They are often used in IVF treatments as they are thought to result in more mature eggs because they stop the release of LH which can cause the follicles to release the eggs before they are ready. Side effects include headaches, mood swings, vaginal dryness and insomnia.

FERTILITY DRUGS FOR MEN If there are problems with the quality and quantity of your partner's sperm the drugs he may be offered include:

~ *hCG and hMG:* these can be used separately or together for men with low levels of LH and FSH, which in turn can cause problems with sperm production.
~ *Bromocriptine:* men who have high levels of prolactin, which can cause loss of libido and impotence, may be offered this prolactin-lowering drug.
~ *Clomiphene or tamoxifen:* these are both anti-oestrogens which have been given to men with low sperm count or who have hormonal imbalance but their value remains questionable. Testosterone is another fertility treatment in which there is no evidence of effectiveness.
~ *Corticosteroids:* these are sometimes used for men who have antisperm antibodies but again there isn't enough evidence for their effectiveness. Side effects include weight gain, bloating, rashes and insomnia.

ASSISTED-CONCEPTION TECHNIQUES

SUCCESS FOR IVF – UK DATA FOR 2003/2004

Below 35 years 27.6%

35–37 . . . . 23.3%

38–39 . . . . 18.3%

40–42 . . . . 10%

Total 23.1%

INTRA-UTERINE INSEMINATION (IUI)

Also known as artificial insemination, IUI gives sperm a head start by putting it directly into the womb at the time of ovulation to fertilise the egg. In other words, it shortens the distance between egg and sperm and so increases your chances of conceiving.

IUI is less invasive and less expensive than other methods of assisted conception. So, if your diagnosis is one of unexplained infertility, you are under the age of 35 and there is no medical or physical reason why you can't get pregnant, IUI should be the first assisted-conception treatment to consider.

IUI can be used if you have problems with ovulation because stimulating drugs can be given at the same time to increase the chances of its working. It is also suitable if your partner is producing an antisperm antibody (in the sperm only, not in the blood), which means his sperm will not penetrate your cervical mucus.

This form of treatment is not appropriate for women with blocked or damaged fallopian tubes, poor egg quality or for women aged over 40.

What happens?

You and your partner will need to go to the clinic around the time you are ovulating and your partner will be asked to provide a fresh semen sample. Ultrasound is then used to track the development of the follicles so that sperm can be inserted high into your womb at ovulation through a fine catheter. IUI can feel embarrassing and a little uncomfortable but it is not painful. No anaesthetic is needed and you will have to rest for a while afterwards.

Success rate

Success rates for IUI are between 10 and 15 per cent per cycle. Success depends on the age of the woman, the quality of the sperm and how long a couple have been trying.

Unfortunately, it isn't offered enough in my opinion and too many clinics jump straight to IVF treatments; perhaps because they are more lucrative than IUI which costs far less.

IN-VITRO FERTILISATION (IVF)

IVF involves fertilising a woman's eggs outside her body under controlled laboratory conditions – hence the phrase 'test-tube baby' – then placing the fertilised egg back into her womb.

IVF is by far the most popular method of assisted conception. Although originally designed for women with fallopian tube damage, it is now used for couples with a wide range of fertility problems, including abnormal sperm, ovulation problems, endometriosis and unexplained infertility.

What happens?

To prepare your body for IVF, GnRH analogues are given, either via a nasal spray or daily injection, putting your body into a temporary menopausal state so that your own hormones won't interfere with the treatment. Another fertility drug, FSH or hMG, is then given via injections to stimulate several follicles to develop and once there are enough follicles of the correct size (as monitored by ultrasound) an injection of HcG will be given which primes the eggs before they are collected. About 36 hours later the eggs are collected through the vagina using an aspiration needle guided by ultrasound. The aim is to collect about 20 eggs. During this procedure you may be sedated or given a general anaesthetic.

Meanwhile your partner will be required to supply a fresh semen sample, if necessary 'washed' in a special fluid so that the weaker sperm are filtered out. (Sperm washing, or quality control, may also be a feature of IUI treatment.) The sperm is then mixed with each egg and those that are fertilised and dividing well will be chosen to go back into the womb. This takes place about two or three days later and the embryos are transferred into the womb via the cervix, using a soft catheter. A maximum of two embryos can be implanted according to UK law (this is likely to be reduced to one, except in 'older' women) and the hope is that they will implant into the womb within seven to eight days. In order to increase the chances of implantation, the hormone progesterone is given either as pessaries or injections.

Success rate

Success rates do vary throughout the country and in different countries, but as you can see from the table above the average 15 to 25 per cent success rate of IVF is lower than all the hype might suggest. IVF treatment most commonly fails during the implantation stage. Sometimes the IVF cycle is abandoned because the drugs aren't stimulating the eggs or because they are stimulating them too much, causing hyperstimulation which is potentially dangerous. Bear in mind too that although fertility clinics follow the same IVF process they also apply their own variations to increase the chances of success.

The risk of multiple births, not surprisingly, increases with IVF treatment which is why according to UK law only two embryos can be transferred in any one treatment cycle for women under 40 and no more than three in women over 40. In the USA such regulations are not always in place but seeing as a number of European studies also indicate that transferring multiple embryos depletes the nutritional environment in the uterus, it really does make good medical and reproductive sense to keep the number of embryos transferred to a minimum.[7]

GAMETE INTRA FALLOPIAN TRANSFER (GIFT)

Although fairly popular in the 1980s and '90s, GIFT is now being used much less frequently than IVF. In this procedure your eggs are mixed (not fertilised) with your partner's sperm in a dish and then put back into the fallopian tubes so that fertilisation takes place where it should happen naturally. GIFT is only suitable for women with healthy fallopian tubes.

What happens?
The use of drugs is identical to IVF but the difference is that egg retrieval is done by a laparoscope (telescope) through the abdomen and so a general anaesthetic is needed (which is probably what has made it less popular). A maximum of three eggs are put back into the fallopian tubes. The main difference between GIFT and IVF is that fertilisation takes place inside the body, but it is also more invasive and expensive.

Success rate
To date there are no success rates for GIFT because it does not come under the HFEA (Human Fertilisation and Embryo Authority) which only monitors techniques involving an embryo outside the body. Some clinics, however, believe that GIFT is more successful than IVF because fertilisation takes place where nature intended, i.e. in the fallopian tubes.

GIFT-ET

GIFT-ET is another technique that seemed to be popular for a while and is not used very much now. It involved a combination of GIFT and IVF, with both procedures performed in the same cycle. One or two eggs are collected and mixed with sperm and but back into the fallopian tubes and, at the same time, one fertilised egg is put back into the womb. As with GIFT a woman's fallopian tubes must be healthy for this option to be considered and a general anaesthetic is used.

MICROMANIPULATION TECHNIQUES

Once sperm and egg have been collected, the embryologist may decide to increase your chances of successful fertilisation by assisting the egg and or sperm in some way. These techniques are called micromanipulation methods and include ICSI and assisted hatching.

Intracytoplasmic sperm injection (ICSI)

This treatment involves a single sperm being injected directly into the egg to fertilise it and the embryo then being implanted into the womb. ICSI can be used if your partner's sperm count is so low that IVF is not viable, if he cannot ejaculate or if he has an obstruction preventing release of his sperm.

For ICSI you undergo the same drug preparation as with IVF. The success rate for ICSI is slightly higher than for IVF (25–30 per cent). In men who can't ejaculate or whose sperm is obstructed the sperm samples can be drawn off directly from the testes but if this doesn't work a biopsy is performed, in which fingernail-sized pieces are taken from the testes through a tiny incision.

Medically, for male factor fertility, ICSI is usually the only solution. This means that for couples where the woman does not have a fertility problem but her partner does, she would have to go through an ICSI treatment with the drug protocols in order to get pregnant. So it is definitely worth it for couples – especially the man, in this case – to follow the fertility-boosting recommendations in this book because if it is just low sperm count or high abnormal sperm that is the problem, you may find that after three months you might not need an ICSI treatment after all.

The biggest concern with this treatment is that while in IVF a number of sperm are put in with the egg and the healthiest sperm compete to fertilise it, in ICSI the egg has to accept whatever sperm is inserted. There have been concerns that ICSI can increase the risk of babies born with chromosome defects or having genetic problems later in life. Some men with severe sperm abnormalities (which would be the reason they needed ICSI in the first place) may have an abnormality of the Y chromosome which is likely to be inherited if they have a baby boy. This means that when that boy grows up, he is going to need ICSI in order to conceive with his partner and so the cycle continues. (Before techniques like this were available, men with this abnormality of the Y chromosome would not have been able to conceive and so would not pass the defect on. With the techniques available nowadays we are losing some of the reproductive process's in-built 'survival of the fittest' response.) There have also been reports of an increase in abnormalities of both the X and Y chromosomes in ICSI babies and sometimes these can cause intellectual problems (three times more than would be expected from natural conception).

It has therefore been suggested that men go for genetic testing before they embark on ICIS to rule out any genetic causes of infertility. Counselling should also be offered as if there is a genetic problem they will have to consider that in some cases they are effectively passing on a fertility problem to their children.

In an ICSI treatment cycle poor, weak sperm can be used to fertilise the egg, but in natural conception these weak sperm would never have made the distance. Also in natural conception only the head of the sperm penetrates the egg, while in ICSI the whole of the sperm is injected in. Research has now looked at the risk of developmental problems in babies conceived by this method. One study[8] found that 4.2 per cent of ICSI babies had a malformation which mainly affected the boy's reproductive and urinary systems (three times higher risk than babies conceived naturally). Also the same study showed that babies born by either ICSI or IVF were more likely to have had medical treatment, surgery or a major childhood illness before the age of five.

So the goal is still to help you conceive naturally by following the recommendations in this book. Some of you are going to need an IVF or ICSI treatment, but by putting into place Steps 1 to 5 before embarking on the treatment cycle, you are aiming to get both eggs and sperm as healthy as possible to give you the best chance of a healthy baby and a healthy child with a strong immune system.

Assisted hatching (AH)
In order for an embryo to hatch and attach itself to the lining of the womb, a small hole is made, during natural conception, in the casing (zona pellucida) of the embryo. In natural conception, enzymes present in the fallopian tube help to soften the casing as the fertilised egg travels down into the womb. This is obviously bypassed in IVF and ICSI because the embryos are placed directly into the womb. However, a technique called assisted hatching can be used to make a hole artificially with either a laser or chemical to aid hatching and implantation. Assisted hatching was often used for 'older' women in whom the zona pellucida can be harder and for women

who have produced good-quality eggs in an IVF cycle but in whom implantation has not occurred.

In 2003, the National Institute for Clinical Excellence (NICE) Fertility Guideline recommended that 'assisted hatching should not be offered because it has not been shown to be effective in increasing pregnancy rates'. A review of the literature showed that assisted hatching does improve the implantation rates in younger women and in those women have had previous unsuccessful IVF cycles, but who ironically, did not improve the chances of an older woman (over 35) achieving a pregnancy. Not many clinics still do assisted hatching.

Surgical aspiration of sperm

If no sperm is found in your partner's semen, due to infections or physical problems, sperm can be aspirated surgically from the epididymis (the fine tubule of the testicle) in a procedure known as sperm aspiration, performed under a general anaesthetic. The couple would then have an ICSI cycle.

PGD (pre-implantation genetic diagnosis)

You may have been screened for genetic diseases and found that there is a problem. In PGD, one or two cells are removed from the developing embryos and tested for genetic diseases and embryos that do not have the genes for that problem are then chosen to be used in that cycle of IVF or ICSI.

EMBRYO TRANSFER

Embryos that occur as a result of IVF and ICSI are transferred into your womb between two and five days after egg collection. On a daily basis after collection they will be monitored for cell division and you will be told how many have fertilised successfully. Each day the embryologist will be looking for steady advancement in cell division and based on daily observation and monitoring he or she will decide which is the ideal day for embryo transfer to take place.

Once five days have passed the embryo will be at a developmental stage known as blastocyst and day five transfers are called 'blastocyst transfers'. A blastocyst transfer shows that a number of your embryos are developing healthily and your specialist has the opportunity to choose which are the best candidates. A blastocyst transfer is thought to increase chances of pregnancy by up to 15 per cent.

If a number of healthy embryos remain unused, you may want to freeze them for use in the future. You would not then need a full-blown IVF cycle as ovulation stimulation and egg collection wouldn't be required. Not all embryos survive the thawing process and the success rate is lower than fresh cycles but an estimated 20,000 babies in the UK have been born using frozen, thawed embryos.

Once the embryos have been transferred successfully into your womb via a soft, fine catheter (a relatively painless procedure which takes 20 to 30 minutes) you are free to leave the clinic when you feel ready.

A number of clinics recommend drinking large quantities of milk in order to get enough protein and liquid during IVF or ICSI. Milk is high in saturated fat and nowadays, with intensive milk production, it can also contain high amounts of oestrogen. My suggestion would be to drink plenty of water and herb teas and use other good-quality protein like fish, organic eggs, nuts and seeds. The other benefit of good amounts of protein and liquid during IVF is that it can help to reduce the risk of OHSS (ovarian hyper-stimulation syndrome) where you actually grow too many follicles. The condition causes a shift of fluid and protein balance in the body, the ovaries become greatly enlarged and fluid builds up in the abdomen. The best thing you can do to help yourself during the whole treatment cycle is to get plenty of rest, drink plenty of water and make sure you are getting enough quality protein to produce a good quantity of eggs, encourage embryo development and the implantation process.

COPING WITH THE TWO-WEEK WAIT

If you've been following my boost-your-fertility diet and lifestyle guidelines you will be in good reproductive health, so over the two weeks while you wait to find out if you are pregnant you need to relax as much as you can and, if possible, stop worrying.

In addition to eating healthily and drinking lots of water don't jump back into a hectic lifestyle after embryo transfer. Take it easy and get as much rest and relaxation as you can. You may find that complementary therapies such as acupuncture, meditation or aromatherapy or even simply writing your thoughts and feelings down will help you to stay calm and focused.

Fourteen days can seem like for ever when you are waiting to do a pregnancy test. Avoid buying over-the-counter pregnancy test kits because if used before day 14 they can produce a negative result. The IVF clinic will organise a blood test to show if you actually are pregnant.

When the two weeks are up, if your pregnancy test is positive, you are pregnant and that is wonderful news. Although this is an incredibly happy time, it is only natural to feel anxious and to have fears about losing your pregnancy. The next 12 weeks are crucial for the healthy development of your baby so continue to take it easy and eat well. Stay as positive and upbeat as you can and don't forget to keep taking your supplements. Take fertility multivitamins and minerals containing folic acid (Fertility Plus for Women) for the first three months, then switch to a good antenatal supplement (the one I use in the clinic is called Ante-Natal Plus). You should still take your Vitamin C Plus and Omega 3 Plus fish oil (or linseed oil) unless you are on blood thinners, like aspirin or heparin.

If the test result is negative and you are not pregnant, don't try to hide your feelings of sadness and loss. It is important to acknowledge your loss and to take things one day at a time. Gather support from loved ones or use the counselling services that your fertility clinic can offer you to help you deal with the disappointment and find ways to move on.

WHAT IS A CHEMICAL PREGNANCY? A chemical pregnancy is the term given to a pregnancy that ends very early in the first trimester, typically within the first six weeks. They are confirmed by testing for hCG, the hormones that indicate the presence of a pregnancy. It is believed that chemical pregnancies occur when the foetus dies immediately after conception. This happens before the embryo has a chance to implant properly in your womb where it can grow and develop.

Chemical pregnancies are actually quite common. In fact, between 50 and 60 per cent of all first-time pregnancies are thought to end in miscarriage and a large majority of these can be attributed to chemical pregnancies. Fortunately, the vast majority of women who experience a chemical pregnancy go on to have happy and healthy pregnancies thereafter. In fact, the chances of experiencing multiple chemical pregnancies are quite slim. However, if you have suffered from two or more, it could be a sign of an underlying reproductive problem, so be sure to have further investigations.

SPERM/EGG AND EMBRYO DONATION

IVF treatments can be performed with a couple's own eggs and sperm, but if this is not possible – whether because there is a problem with your partner's sperm or with your eggs or if you have a genetic disease that can be passed on to your baby – there is the option of donor eggs, sperm or embryos to consider.

For men with poor sperm quality or men who have had a vasectomy sperm donation is an option. It is also an option for single women or lesbian couples. Sperm is typically supplied by an anonymous donor aged between 18 and 45 who has been screened for infections and genetic diseases. If a woman is under the age of 30, there is a 13.5 per cent chance of having a baby with donor insemination but after the age of 40 this lowers dramatically to only 2.5 per cent. If you are considering this option bear in mind that in 2005 the legal position changed regarding donor anonymity so that children from donations now have access to information concerning their genetic origins. This will include the donor's name, address, date of birth, district of birth and appearance. Anyone born from donor insemination now has a right to find out this information from the HFEA once they reach the age of 18.

Egg donation is suitable for women who are in menopause, who have no ovaries, who have become infertile due to an illness like cancer or who have had many unsuccessful attempts at IVF because they are unable to produce viable eggs. Success rates for egg donation are higher than IVF at 25–40 per cent as most egg donors tend to be under the age of 35.

If neither the man's sperm nor the woman's eggs can be used, embryo donation is an option to consider. Donated embryos often come from IVF couples who have spare embryos following a successful IVF cycle.

NATURAL IVF

Like standard IVF, natural IVF can help women with blocked or damaged fallopian tubes, or endometriosis, men with low-quality sperm or who suffer with impotency or premature ejaculation and couples with unexplained infertility.

Whereas in standard IVF, drugs are used to stimulate a woman's ovaries to mature more eggs than normal, in a natural IVF cycle the egg is removed just as it is ready to ripen and (as with conventional IVF) it is introduced to the sperm in a Petri dish.

Once fertilised, it is implanted in the womb. Drugs are used only to block the egg ovulating before it is harvested. This method is thought to be particularly helpful when treating older women whose ovaries are more fragile and need gentler handling.

A more natural approach is likely to yield better-quality eggs and reduce the risk of abnormalities, which results in embryos failing to implant or to miscarriages. Natural IVF also means women can have treatments over consecutive months, whereas with standard IVF three-month breaks should be recommended because of the drug regime. Finally, natural IVF is at least three times cheaper.

On the down side, success rates for natural IVF are not as high as with standard IVF. Success rates are 10 per cent per cycle compared with an average of 25 per cent with standard. Also, it may take a number of attempts to retrieve that one egg that is released that month which has then got to fertilise and divide well to be transferred back. In standard IVF many eggs are produced, giving the specialist much more choice of eggs and then embryos.

IMPROVING THE ODDS OF YOUR IVF

Undoubtedly much of the success of your IVF is determined by the quantity and quality of your eggs and your partner's sperm. But there are many things you can do to help improve your odds of getting and staying pregnant.

First and foremost make sure you continue to follow Steps 1 to 4; it is especially important to keep taking your multivitamin and mineral supplements, including folic acid. Don't do anything strenuous, take gentle exercise and stay away from alcohol, caffeine and cigarette smoke.

OUR STORY I am 30 and had a history of flooding and clots each month. I was born with only one ovary and the fallopian tube was slightly twisted. Before coming to the clinic, I had had two myomectomies to remove fibroids and polyps. My husband and I had been trying for a baby for two and a half years with no success and I'd already had one unsuccessful IVF cycle and then an unsuccessful frozen embryo transfer (FET). A month after the FET, I had another myomectomy to remove a large polyp and a couple of smaller fibroids. It was no wonder the FET did not work. My gynaecologist was very keen for me to try IVF again but I was very unhappy about this as the bleeding had started again. Although we wanted a baby, my desire for the monthly flooding to stop was stronger as it was affecting my life.

I had already been following your dietary recommendations and I really enjoyed the diet and actually lost two stone, even though I felt like I was eating lots. I decided to take time out of fertility treatment as I was fed up all the IVF drugs (and before the IVF I had been on clomiphene, tranexamic acid etc.). I came to your clinic in London in January and you recommended the Fertility Plus supplements for both my husband and me. Our hair mineral tests showed that we were both deficient in zinc. You devised a supplement plan for us and I also took the herbs you suggested. As I had intimated that I only wanted to try IVF one more time you suggested that I wait six months and follow the plan.

Within a couple of months of following your plan the bleeding had eased. We started the IVF in June of that same year and I responded extremely well to the treatment. Despite only having one ovary they collected 16 eggs, five of which actually made it to blastocyst stage (obviously my husband's vitamins and diet change had also helped). I had two embryos put back in and on July 4 had a positive pregnancy test. We both truly believe that had we not come to the clinic we would not be expecting this baby now. Your recommendations are so unintrusive and only have the side effects of making you healthy. Before I got pregnant, after following your diet plan and taking the supplements, I looked so much better than I had for years. I was a healthy 10 stone (I am 5' 7") and my hair/ skin/nails look fantastic. So thank you for your advice – I will be eternally grateful.

After the embryos are transferred into your womb and you return home, try and get as much rest as possible, even taking two to three days off work if you can, resting in bed. If that isn't possible, and it won't be for everyone, resume your normal activities in a gentle, calm way. Plenty of rest and a non-stressful environment will boost your chances of conception.

COMPLEMENTARY THERAPIES DURING ASSISTED CONCEPTION I believe, and research can back this up,[9] that gentle therapies such as acupuncture, reflexology, homeopathy, hypnotherapy and relaxation techniques can safely and effectively be used alongside fertility treatments to maximise your chances of success. Do make sure, though, that you work with a qualified practitioner. For more information on which ones to try, see pages 72–76.

THE DARK SIDE OF FERTILITY TREATMENTS

IVF treatments are a modern medicine success story that can help couples who are otherwise unable to have a baby. However, there is a dark side to fertility treatments as well.

All the media hype and focus on the success of IVF means that many couples often have unrealistic expectations. As the statistics show IVF is not a miracle cure for infertility and failure rates are still high (at 75 per cent, if not more, depending on age). And for those who go through the physical trauma (the process is invasive and hard on the woman's body with the drug regime) only to end up with no baby, it is extremely hard to deal with both physically and emotionally. The whole process can place an incredible strain on a relationship and sex can lose its spontaneity and intimacy. It is also important to understand that IVF places unnatural demands upon your body because it is being made to mature a large number of eggs in one cycle, when normally one or two at the most would be released at a time. The big question often asked is what are the long-term effects of taking these drugs on you and the baby that is conceived?

As far as the health and well-being of children born through IVF are concerned, this question is not easily answered. The IVF generation is still growing up and we don't yet know how these drugs will affect their fertility and long-term health. It seems obvious though that unnaturally overstimulating the ovaries with drugs, like clomiphene, may have short- and long-term effects on the mother. Most drugs used to induce ovulation have unpleasant side effects (see page 179).

The harsh reality is that there are still glaring gaps in our knowledge about the dangers that fertility techniques and drugs may pose. Yet I do understand that for many couples it is going to be their only way of having a baby. So that is why I – together with my team of nutritionists – take an integrated approach to fertility. Couples who get into optimum health *before* IVF may manage either to avoid it altogether, succeed with a minimally invasive technique (like IUI) or be successful on the first cycle of IVF. Also by having the right support through IVF, it is possible to minimise the side effects and to increase the chances of having a healthy baby.

WHEN TO CLOSE THE DOOR ON TREATMENT

A decision of how far you are prepared to go with your treatment always has to be made. If you are an NHS patient in the UK, funding may determine the limit. If you are paying for yourself most clinics recommend four treatments with IVF. If you want to keep trying much depends on how much your body, mind and relationship can endure, but it is important that you and your partner always remember that you have a choice and that you recognise your limit. This is different for everyone, but it needs courage to acknowledge when you have reached it.

Some couples start planning for alternatives early on in medical treatment and when they reach their limit, they are prepared to try something else. Agreeing on a limit or time frame is helpful – give yourselves a date when you will discontinue treatment, even if you decide to modify it later.

Another measure that might be useful is to take a short break from treatment. Depending on your feelings after this, you may find that you don't want to continue or that you need to keep going for a while longer.

Infertility treatment with its tests, treatments and endless waiting for results may well have taken over your life, so if you are considering stopping be sure to talk to your partner and/or arrange for sessions with an infertility counsellor. This will help you to let go of your feelings of disappointment and grief and replace them with resolution, closure and a new reality.

OTHER OPTIONS FOR PARENTHOOD

Not being able to have your own children doesn't mean you can't include children in your life. If you feel you need to experience mothering and you and your partner agree that this is something you want to look at, adoption and fostering offer you the chance to raise children. You can make an incredible impact on their lives by teaching, mentoring and role modelling. You don't have to look far to find a child who can benefit from your time and attention, and you should not underestimate the impact that this can have on the life of a child.

Shaping a successful social life can be hard if you are surrounded by people with children and if this causes you pain, seek out those who are living happy and positive child-free lives and get to know them. The number of child-free couples is increasing every year and in the UK ISSUE has set up an organisation for child-free couples called More to Life.

It is important to note that I have used the term child-free rather than childless. This is because more and more couples are making a life choice *not* to have children even if they can. So, when you are ready, perhaps it is time for you to start thinking about the advantages of being child-free, the most significant of these being your freedom – freedom to pursue your interests, career or vocation. Perhaps you will travel or perhaps you will find other ways to parent. You can nurture other people, siblings, friends, parents, godchildren, ideas, communities, projects, jobs, plants, animals and so on.

Whatever you decide, remember that child-free living does not have to be merely tolerated; it can be a positive, fulfilling and joyful experience. And remember also, whenever one door shuts in your life, no amount of tears or anger will open it, but there are always other doors that you can open. Why not see what opportunities, challenges and possibilities are on the other side?

appendix

ANATOMY OF THE FEMALE REPRODUCTIVE SYSTEM

While most women know the basics, many don't realise that there is more to your reproductive system than just your periods, and understanding it is an important part of knowing how to prevent or increase your chances of pregnancy.

THE FEMALE REPRODUCTIVE ORGANS

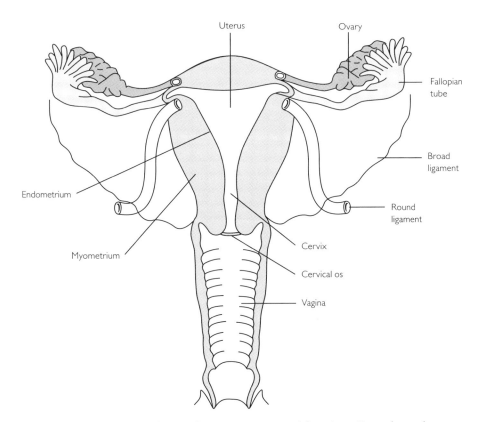

Your reproductive system is designed to carry out several functions. It produces the female egg cells necessary for reproduction (ova or oocytes) and transports the egg to the site of fertilisation. Conception (fertilisation of an egg by a sperm) normally occurs in the fallopian tubes. After fertilisation, the womb offers a safe environment for a baby to develop before it is time for it to make its way into the outside world. If fertilisation does not take place, menstruation follows (the monthly shedding of the womb lining). In addition, the female reproductive system produces the female sex hormones that maintain it. During the menopause the woman literally runs out of eggs and gradually the ovaries stop producing oestrogen.

Your reproductive organs are comprised of a vagina, a cervix, a uterus, fallopian tubes and ovaries. All these organs work together to help you menstruate, conceive and carry a baby to term.

THE VAGINA

The vagina is the canal that joins the cervix (the lower part of womb) to the outside of the body. It is also known as the birth canal and connects your internal reproductive organs with your external genitalia. It ends at the cervix and is the point of entry for the penis to ejaculate sperm during sex, as well as the final passageway through which a baby exits when it is born.

THE CERVIX

Situated between the vagina and womb, the cervix secretes mucus that can help or obstruct sperm in fertilising an egg. It is the opening through which sperm must pass in order to get to the egg. A baby must also go through the cervix as it exits the womb and enters the vagina.

THE UTERUS

The uterus (or womb) is a hollow, pear-shaped organ located at the base of the pelvic cavity. It is home to a developing baby (foetus) and protects and nourishes the foetus until birth. The womb is divided into two parts: the cervix (see above) and the main body of the uterus, called the corpus. The corpus can easily expand to hold a developing baby. The uterine lining, known as the endometrium, builds up during the luteal phase of the menstrual cycle (see page 199) in preparation for an embryo from the fallopian tube. If there is no pregnancy it is shed as menstrual blood during menstruation.

THE FALLOPIAN TUBES

These are narrow tubes attached to the upper part of the uterus and serve as tunnels for the ova (egg) to travel from the ovaries to the womb. They have 20–25 finger-like structures on their ends that hover just above the ovaries and work to collect the mature egg when it is released and push the egg down; if the egg meets sperm coming up the tube, fertilisation can take place. Conception, the fertilisation of an egg by a sperm, normally occurs in the fallopian tubes. The fertilised embryo then moves to the womb, where it implants in the womb lining. If the fallopian tubes are damaged or blocked the embryo won't be able to travel and may implant in the fallopian tube. This is called an ectopic pregnancy and is potentially life threatening; surgery to remove the embryo and in some cases part of the fallopian tube in which it has implanted is required.

THE OVARIES

The ovaries are small, oval glands about the size of walnuts, located on either side of the uterus just below the fallopian tubes. Women usually have two ovaries, one on each side of the womb. Ovaries are the storing house for fluid-filled sacs called egg follicles; every month, one of these egg follicles will mature and release an egg which is picked up by the fallopian tube. The ovaries are also responsible for producing oestrogen and progesterone, which are vital for proper reproductive function. At birth, there are approximately 1 million eggs; and by the time of puberty, only about 400,000 remain. The rate of loss continues until they are depleted at menopause, typically around the age of 50–52.

WHAT HAPPENS DURING THE MENSTRUAL CYCLE?

FEMALE HORMONAL PANEL

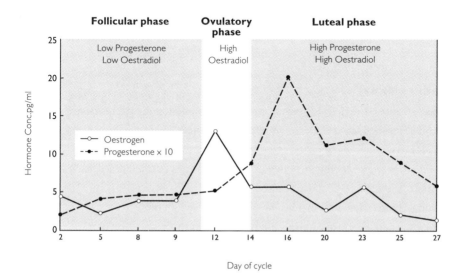

Day of cycle

Women of reproductive age experience cycles of hormonal activity that repeat at about one-month intervals. With every cycle, a woman's body prepares for a potential pregnancy, whether or not that is her intention. The term menstruation refers to the periodic shedding of the womb lining.

The average menstrual cycle takes about 28 days and occurs in phases: the follicular, ovulatory (ovulation) and the luteal phases. There are four major hormones involved in the menstrual cycle: follicle-stimulating hormone (FSH), luteinising hormone (LH), oestrogen (oestradiol) and progesterone.

A NORMAL FEMALE HORMONAL CYCLE

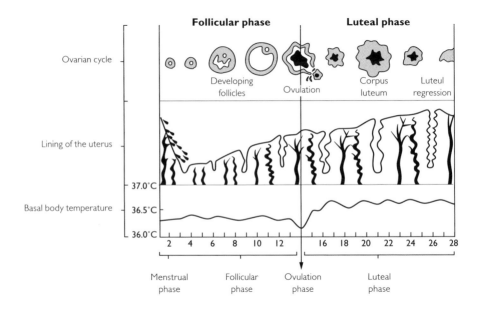

FOLLICULAR PHASE

This phase starts on the first day of your period and the following events occur:

~ FSH and LH are released from the pituitary gland in the brain and travel in the blood to the ovaries.

~ The hormones stimulate the growth of about 15–20 eggs in the ovaries, each in its own 'shell' or follicle.

~ FSH and LH also trigger an increase in oestrogen production.

~ As the oestrogen level rises, like a switch, it turns off the production of FSH. This careful balance of hormones allows the body to limit the number of follicles that complete maturation, or growth.

~ As the follicular phase progresses, one follicle in one ovary becomes dominant and
continues to mature, suppressing all the other follicles in the group which stop
growing and die. The dominant follicle continues to produce oestrogen.

OVULATORY PHASE

The ovulatory phase, or ovulation, starts about 10–14 days after the follicular phase
started. It is the midpoint of the menstrual cycle, with the next menstrual period
starting about two weeks later. During this phase, the following events occur:

~ The rise in oestrogen from the dominant follicle triggers a surge in the amount of LH
produced by the pituitary gland, causing the dominant follicle to release its egg from
the ovary.

~ As the egg is released (ovulation) it is captured by finger-like projections on the end
of the fallopian tubes (fimbriae) which sweep the egg into the tube.

~ There is also an increase in the amount and thickness of mucus produced by the
cervix. In the event of intercourse this thick, stretchy, alkaline mucus can capture
sperm, nourish it, and help it move towards the egg for fertilisation.

LUTEAL PHASE

The luteal phase (second half of the cycle) begins right after ovulation and involves the
following processes:

~ Once it releases its egg, the empty follicle develops into a new structure called the
corpus luteum.

~ The corpus luteum secretes progesterone which prepares the womb for a fertilised
egg to implant.

~ If intercourse has taken place and a man's sperm has fertilised the egg (conception),
the fertilised egg (embryo) will travel through the fallopian tube to implant in the
womb. The woman is now considered pregnant. If the egg is not fertilised, it passes
through the womb. Not needed to support a pregnancy, the lining of the uterus then
breaks down and sheds and the next menstrual period begins.

CONCEPTION AND PREGNANCY

Once an egg has been released from the ovaries, it will begin to travel down the
fallopian tubes towards the womb. As it advances towards the uterus, it begins to
produce an enzyme that helps to attract and guide any sperm that may have been
ejaculated into the female reproductive system during sex.

Although a man releases millions of sperm when he ejaculates during orgasm,
only a few hundred will make it all the way from the cervix up into the uterus and

then into the correct fallopian tube. Just one sperm will then be able to make its way through your egg's tough coating (zona pellucida) to fertilise the egg. The fertilised egg will continue travelling down the fallopian tube and implant itself in the thick womb (endometrial) lining and continue to divide. Your body will also probably start letting you know that it is pregnant.

ANATOMY OF THE MALE REPRODUCTIVE SYSTEM

The main function of the male reproductive system is to produce, nourish and transport sperm and semen, discharge sperm into the female reproductive tract and produce and secrete male reproductive hormones.

THE MALE REPRODUCTIVE ORGANS

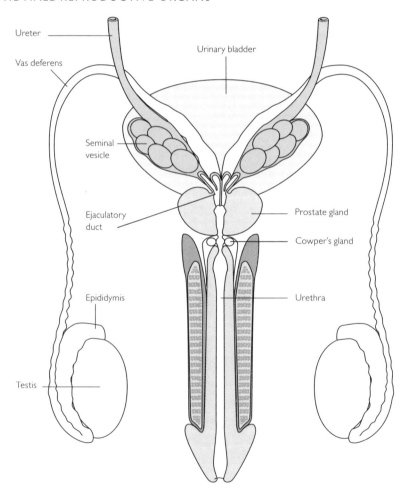

THE PENIS

This is the male organ used in sexual intercourse. At its tip is the opening of the urethra, which transports semen and urine. The body of the penis is cylindrical in shape and consists of circular shaped chambers. These are made up of sponge-like tissue containing thousands of large spaces that fill with blood when the man is sexually aroused. As the penis fills with blood, it becomes rigid and erect, allowing for penetration during sexual intercourse. The skin of the penis is loose and elastic to accommodate changes in penis size during an erection. Semen, which contains sperm (reproductive cells), is expelled (ejaculated) through the end of the penis when the man reaches sexual climax (orgasm). When the penis is erect, the flow of urine is blocked from the urethra, allowing only semen to be ejaculated at orgasm.

SCROTUM

This is the pouch of skin behind the penis that contains the testicles (or testes) and many nerve endings. It is responsible for temperature regulation (sperm development requires a cooler temperature than that of the body) and special muscles in the wall of the scrotum allow it to contract and relax, moving the testicles closer to the body for warmth or further away from the body to cool the temperature.

TESTICLES (TESTES) These are oval organs about the size of large olives that lie in the scrotum, secured at either end by a structure called the spermatic cord. Most men have two testes and they are responsible for making testosterone, the primary male sex hormone, and for generating sperm. Within the testes are coiled masses of tubes called seminiferous tubules, responsible for producing sperm cells.

INTERNAL MALE REPRODUCTIVE ORGANS

Also called accessory organs, these include the following:

Epididymis: a long, coiled tube within the testes which stores and develops the sperm cells and transfers mature ones into the vas deferens (see below). During sexual arousal, contractions force the sperm into the vas deferens.
Vas deferens: a long, muscular tube that carries mature sperm from the epididymis to the urethra in preparation for ejaculation.
Urethra: a tube that carries urine from the bladder and semen during sex to the outside of the body, in preparation for ejaculation.
Seminal vesicles: sac-like pouches that attach to the vas deferens near the base of the bladder which produce a sugar-rich fluid (fructose) providing sperm with a source

of energy to help them move. The fluid of the seminal vesicles makes up most of the volume of a man's ejaculatory fluid, or ejaculate.

Prostate gland: a walnut-sized structure located below the urinary bladder in front of the rectum and which empties into the urethra. It contains prostate fluids that nourish the sperm and provide additional fluid to ejaculate.

HOW THE MALE REPRODUCTIVE SYSTEM WORKS

The primary hormones involved in the male reproductive system are FSH (needed for sperm production), LH (which stimulates the production of testosterone) and testosterone (responsible for male sexual development and sexual arousal). FSH stimulates the production of sperm by Sertoli cells and spermatids (basically immature sperm) are embedded in Sertoli cells and develop into sperm (spermatogenesis). A high FSH level in a man can indicate that his body is struggling to produce sperm.

Beginning at puberty the testicles typically produce around 50,000 new sperm every minute of the day and this continues until a man is 70 or older. Each sperm cell consists of a head (acrosome) which carries one half a man's genetic code – 23 chromosomes, a mid-portion, the energy powerhouse and a tail (flagella) which help the sperm swim to and penetrate the egg.

Sperm development and cell division which produces mature sperm occurs in the seminiferous tubules and one sperm takes about 100 days or three months to develop. That's why it's so important for your partner to allow three to four months for their pre-conception diet and lifestyle plan (Steps 1 to 4) before trying to conceive.

When almost mature, sperm leave the tubules and move along the fine tubes of the epididymis to complete their development into fully mature sperm. During this part of their journey they will move into the vas deferens, wait for muscular contractions and sexual arousal and combine with the fluid from the prostate gland before ejaculating through the urethra. Each ejaculate contains up to 300 million sperm, but only 1 million reach the cervix, 200 reach the fallopian tube and one fertilises an egg. Within ten minutes of reaching the vagina the sperm enter the uterus swimming at a speed of 2–3mm per minute. The fittest and healthiest sperm usually reach the fallopian tube within two hours.

FERTILISATION AND IMPLANTATION

As few as fifty sperm reach the egg and only one will eventually penetrate it. The penetrating sperm must shed a protein coating from its head and release enzymes before it can pass through the ovum's protective layers. Normally, once a sperm has made its way into the egg, the ovum will automatically prevent other sperm from entering.

Fertilisation takes place at the upper end of the fallopian tubes, but the fertilised egg must be implanted into the womb lining where it can receive nourishment and oxygen. The first cell division takes place within 12 hours of fertilisation. For the three days following fertilisation, the egg will move towards the uterus, growing all the time.

By the fourth day after fertilisation, the egg is about the size of a small blackberry and is ready for implantation. To be implanted, the fertilised egg must shed its shell (it then becomes known as the blastocyst) and 'burrow' into the lining of the uterus. Once implanted, the blastocyst begins to develop into an embryo. Successful implantation has the effect of releasing hCG (human chorionic gonadotrophin) to maintain the pregnancy – hCG is the hormone detected in pregnancy tests. Progesterone and oestrogen levels continue to rise for up to three months after implantation to ensure the continuation of the pregnancy until the placenta takes over at about 12–14 weeks. At the end of the 40-week 'gestation' or growth period, a baby is born.

REFERENCES

USING THIS BOOK

1 National Statistics, http://www.statistics.gov.uk/pdfdir/poptrd0305.pdf

2 The National Women's Health Study, 2004, `Assembly and description of a population-based reproductive cohort', *Bioorganic and Medical Chemistry Public Health*, Aug 7, 4, 35.

3 Dunson, B. *et al*, 2004, `Increased infertility with age in men and women', *Obstetrics and Gynaecology*. Jan, 103(1), 51–56.

4 Hassan, M. *et al*, 2004, `Negative lifestyle is associated with a significant reduction in fecundity', *Fertility and Sterility*, Feb, 81(2), 384–392.

5 Ontario Early Child Development Research Centre Preconception and Health: Research and strategies: Best start brochure 2001.

6 Oliva, A. *et al*, 2001, `Contribution of environmental factors to the risk of male infertility', *Human Reproduction*, 16, 8, Aug.

7 Dunlop, A.L. *et al*, 2007, `National recommendations for preconception care: The essential role of the family physician', *Journal of the American Board of Family Medicine*, Jan–Feb, 20(1), 81–84; Grainger, D.A. *et al*, 2006, `Preconception care and treatment with assisted reproductive technologies', *Maternal and Child Health Journal*, Sep, 10(5 Suppl), S161–164; Cikot, R. *et al*, 1999, `Dutch GPs acknowledge the need for preconceptual health care', *British Journal of General Practice*, Apr, 49(441), 314; Posner, S.F. *et al*, 2006, `The national summit on preconception care: a summary of concepts and recommendations', *Maternal and Child Health Journal*, Sep, 10(5 Suppl), S197–205.

8 `Changing unhealthy habits. Essential step to a healthier life', *Mayo Clinic Health Letter*, 2007, Feb, Suppl, 1–8.

STEP ONE YOUR DIET

1 Hoare, J. *et al*, 1999, `The National Diet and Nutrition Survey: adults aged 19–64 years', *Volume 5 Summary Report*, HMSO, London.

2 Simopoulos, A., 1991, `Omega 3 fatty acids in health and disease and in growth and development', *American Journal of Clinical Nutrition*, 54, 438–463.

3 Lobstein, T., 2005, 'Plants lose their value', *The Food Magazine*, 68, 12-13.

4 Swan, S. *et al*, 1998, `A prospective study of spontaneous abortion: relation to amount and source of drinking water consumed in early pregnancy', *Epidemiology*, Mar, 9(2), 126–133.

5 Marsh, K. *et al*, 2005, `The optimal diet for women with polycystic ovary syndrome', *British Journal of Nutrition*, Aug, 94(2), 154–165.

6 Maconochie, N. *et al*, 2007, `Risk factors for first trimester miscarriage – results from a UK-population-based case-control study', *British Journal of General Practice*, Feb, 114(2), 170–186.

7 Vander, W. *et al*, 2005, `Short-term effect of eggs on satiety in overweight and obese subjects', *Journal of the American College of Nutrition*, Dec, 24(6), 510–515.

8 Cho, E. *et al*, 2006, *Archives of Internal Medicine*, 166, 2253–2259.

9 Parazzini, F. *et al*, 2004, `Selected food intake and risk of endometriosis', *Human Reproduction*, Aug, 19(8), 1755–1759. Epub 2004 Jul 14.

10 Steck, S.E. *et al*, 2007, `Cooked meat and risk of breast cancer – lifetime versus recent dietary intake', *Epidemiology*, May, 18(3), 373–382.

11 Greenlee, A.R. *et al*, 2003, `Risk factors for female infertility in an agricultural region', *Epidemiology*, Jul, 14(4), 429–436.

12 Cramner, D. *et al*, 1994, `Adult hypolactasia, milk consumption, and age-specific fertility', *American Journal of Epidemiology*, Feb 1, 139(3), 282–289.

13 Nagata, C. *et al*, 2000, 'Inverse association of soy product intake with serum androgen and estrogen concentrations in Japanese men', *Nutrition and Cancer*, 38, 37–39.

14 Chavarro, J. *et al*, 2007, `A prospective study of dairy foods intake and anovulatory infertility', *Human Reproduction*, May, 22(5), 1340–1347. Epub 2007 Feb 28.

15 Xu, Y. *et al*, 2007, `Effect of placental fatty acid metabolism and regulation by peroxisome proliferator activated receptor on pregnancy and fetal outcomes', *Journal of Pharmaceutical Sciences*, 96(10), 2582–2606.

16 Chavarro, J. *et al*, 2007, `Dietary fatty acid intakes and the risk of ovulatory infertility', *American Journal of Clinical Nutrition*, Jan, 85(1), 231.

17 Myers, G. *et al*, 2007, `Maternal fish consumption benefits children's development', *Lancet*, Feb 17,

369(9561), 537–538.

[18] Daniels, J.L. *et al*, 2005, `Fish intake during pregnancy and early cognitive development of offspring', *Obstetrical and Gynaecological Survey*, 60, 80–81; 2007, `Experts say benefits of eating fish outweigh possible risks', *Harvard Women's Health Watch*, Feb 14(6), 6–7.

[19] Xue, F. *et al*, 2007, `Maternal fish consumption, mercury levels, and risk of preterm delivery', *Environmental Health Perspectives*, Jan, 115(1), 42–47.

[20] Dixon, R. *et al*, 2004, `Phytoestrogens', *Annual Review of Plant Biology*, 55, 225–261.

[21] Jescheke, U. *et al*, 2005, `Effects of phytoestrogens genistein and daidzein on production of human chorionic gonadotropin in term trophoblast cells in vitro', *Gynecological Endocrinology*, Sep, 21(3), 180–184.

[22] West, K. *et al*, 1999, `Double-blind cluster randomized trial of low-dose supplementation with vitamin A or beta-carotene on mortality related to pregnancy in Nepal', *British Medical Journal*, 318, 570–575.

[23] Del Bianco, A. *et al*, 2004, `Recurrent spontaneous miscarriages and hyperhomocysteinemia', *Minerva Ginecologica*, Oct, 56(5), 379–383.

[24] Bennet, M. *et al*, 2001, `Vitamin B12 deficiency, infertility and recurrent fetal loss', *Journal of Reproductive Medicine*, Mar, 46(3), 209–212.

[25] Forges, T. *et al*, 2007, `Impact of folate and homocysteine metabolism on human reproductive health', *Human Reproduction Update*, May–Jun, 13(3), 225–238.

[26] Pitkin, R. *et al*, 2007, `Folate and neural tube defects', *American Journal of Clinical Nutrition*, Jan, 85(1), 285S–288S.

[27] Chra, I. *et al*, 2003, `Ascorbic acid and infertility treatment', *Central European Journal of Public Health*, Jun, 11(2), 63–67.

[28] Akman, M. *et al*, 2006, `Improvement in human semen quality after oral supplementation of vitamin C', *Journal of Medicinal Food*, Fall, 9(3), 440–442.

[29] Agarwal, A. *et al*, 2005, `Role of oxidative stress in female reproduction', *Reproductive Biology and Endocrinology*, Jul 14, 3, 28.

[30] Shewita, S. *et al*, 2005, `Mechanisms of male infertility: role of antioxidants', *Current Drug Metabolism*, Oct, 6(5), 495–501.

[31] Ebish, I. *et al*, 2007, `The importance of folate, zinc and antioxidants in the pathogenesis and prevention of subfertility', *Human Reproduction*, 13, 163–174.

[32] Ericson, J. *et al*, 2007, `Prenatal manganese levels linked to childhood behavioural disinhibition', *Neurotoxicology and Teratology*, Mar-Apr, 29(2), 181–187. Epub 2006 Sep 27; Sener, G. *et al*, 1985, `Hair manganese concentrations in newborns and their mothers', *American Journal of Clinical Nutrition*, May, 41(5), 1042–1044. Update, 2007, Mar–Apr, 13(2), 163–174. Epub 2006 Nov 11.

[33] Tod, K. *et al*, 2006, `Selenium and glutathion peroxidase enzyme levels in diabetic patients with early spontaneous abortions', *Akush Ginekol (Sofiia)*, 45(5), 3–9.

[34] Howard, J. *et al*, 1994, `Red cell magnesium and glutathione peroxidase in infertile women – effects of oral supplementation with magnesium and selenium', *Magnesium Research*, Mar, 7(1), 49–57.

[35] Ackmal, M. *et al*, 2006, `Improvement in human semen quality after oral supplementation of vitamin C', *Journal of Medicinal Food*, Fall, 9(3), 440–442; Wang, S. *et al*, 2007, `Beneficial effects of vitamin E in sperm functions in the rat after spinal cord injury', *Journal of Andrology*, Mar–Apr, 28(2), 334–341. Epub 2006 Nov 1; Eskenazi, B. *et al*, 2005, `Antioxidant intake is associated with semen quality in healthy men', *Human Reproduction*, Apr, 20(4), 1006–1012. Epub 2005 Jan 21; Shalini, S. *et al*, 2005, `Role of selenium in regulation of spermatogenesis: involvement of activator protein 1', *BioFactors*, 23(3) 151–162; Tavilian, H. *et al*, 2006, `Decreased polyunsaturated and increased saturated fatty acid concentration in spermatozoa from asthenozoospermic males as compared with normozoospermic males', *Andrologia*, Oct, 38(5), 173–178; Comahire, F. *et al*, 2003, `The role of food supplements in the treatment of the infertile man', *Reproductive BioMedicine Online*, Oct–Nov, 7(4), 385–391.

[36] Wilcox, A. *et al*, 1989, `Caffeinated beverages and decreased fertility', *Lancet*, Apr 15, 1(8642), 840.

[37] Barbieri, R. *et al*, 2001, `The initial fertility consultation: recommendations concerning cigarette smoking, body mass index, and alcohol and caffeine consumption', *American Journal of Obstetrics and Gynecology*, 185(5) 1168–1173.

[38] Nawrt, P. et al, 2003, `Effects of caffeine on human health', Food Additives and Contaminants, Jan, 20(1), 1–30.

[39] Giannelli, M. et al, 2003, `The effect of caffeine consumption and nausea on the risk of miscarriage', Paediatrics Perinatal Epidemiology, 17, 316–323.

[40] Helgstrand, S. et al, 2005, `Maternal underweight and the risk of spontaneous abortion', Acta Obstetrics Gynecology Scandinavia, Dec, 84(12), 1197–2011.

[41] Nelson, S. et al, 2007, `The preconceptual contraception paradigm: obesity and infertility', Humun Reproduction, Apr, 22(4), 912–915. Epub 2006 Dec 15; Gesink, L. et al, 2007, `Obesity and time to pregnancy', Human Reproduction, Feb, 22(2), 414–420. Epub 2006 Nov 9.

[42] Clarm, A. et al, 1995, `Weight Loss results in significant improvement in pregnancy and ovulation rates in annovulatory obese women', Human Reproduction, 10(1), 2705–2712.

[43] Linsten, A. et al, 2005, `Effects of subfertility cause, smoking and body weight on the success rate of IVF', Human Reproduction, Jul, 20(7), 1867–1875. Epub 2005 Apr 7.

[44] Davis, M. et al, 2006, `Evidence for effects of weight on reproduction in women', Reproductive BioMedicine Online, May, 12(5), 552–561; Sarwar, D. et al, 2006, `Pregnancy and obesity: a review and agenda for future research', Journal of Women's Health (Larchmont), Jul–Aug, 15(6), 720–733.

[45] Pirke, K. et al, 1985, `The influence of dieting on the menstrual cycle of healthy young women', Journal of Clinical Endocrinology and Metabolism, 60, 1174–1179.

[46] Rock, C.L. et al, 1996, 'Nutritional characteristics, eating pathology and hormonal status in young women', American Journal of Clinical Nutrition, 64(4), 566–571.

[47] Bates, G. et al, 1982, `Reproductive failure in women who practise weight control', Fertility and Sterility, 37(3), 373–378.

[48] Foreyt, J. et al, 1998, `Obesity, a never ending cycle', International Journal of Fertility and Women's Medicine, 48, 111–116.

[49] Altschuler, J. et al, 2007, `The effect of cinnamon on A1C among adolescents with type 1 diabetes', Diabetes Care, Apr, 30(4), 813–816.

[50] Sallmen, M. et al, 2006, `Reduced fertility among overweight and obese men', Epidemiology, Sep, 17(5), 520–523; Kort, H. et al, 2006, `Impact of body mass index values on sperm quantity and quality', Journal of Andrology, May–Jun, 27(3), 450–452. Epub 2005 Dec 8.

[51] Ramlau-Hansen, C.H. et al, 2007, `Parental infertility and semen quality in male offspring: a follow-up study', American Journal of Epidemiology, 166(5), 568–570, Jun 4.

STEP TWO CHANGING YOUR LIFESTYLE

[1] Hassan, M. et al, 2004, `Negative lifestyle is associated with a significant reduction in fecundity', Fertility and Sterility, 81, 384–392.

[2] Homan, G.F. et al, 2007, `The impact of lifestyle factors on reproductive performance in the general population and those undergoing fertility treatment: a review', Human Reproduction Update, 13(3), 209–223.

[3] Visser, J. et al, 2006, `Anti-mullerian hormone: a new marker for ovarian function', Human Reproduction, 131, 1–9.

[4] La Marca, A. and Volpe A., 2006, `Anti-mullerian hormone in female reproduction: Is measurement of circulating AMH a useful tool?', Clinical Endocrinology, 6, 603–610.

[5] Muttukrishna, S. et al, 2005, `Antral follicle count, anti-mullerian hormone and inhibin B: predictors of ovarian response in assisted reproductive technology?', British Journal of General Practice, 10, 1384–1390.

[6] van Rooij, T.A. et al, 2005, `Serum anti-mullerian hormone levels best reflect the reproductive decline with age in normal women with proven fertility: a longitudinal study', Fertility and Sterility, 83, 979–987.

[7] Maconochie, N. et al, 2007, `Risk factors for first trimester miscarriage – results from a UK-population-based case-control study', British Journal of General Practice, Feb, 114(2), 170–186.

[8] Archer, N. et al, 2007, `Association of paternal age with prevalence of selected birth defects', Birth Defects Research Part A: Clinical and Molecular Teratology, Jan, 79(1), 27–34; Bray, I. et al, 2006, `Advanced paternal age: how old is too old?', Journal of Epidemiology and Community Health, Oct, 60(10), 851–853.

[9] Shew, S. et al, 2005, `Mechanisms of male infertility:

role of antioxidants', *Current Drug Metabolism*, Oct, 6(5), 495–501; Greco, E. *et al*, 2005, `ICSI in cases of sperm DNA damage: beneficial effect of oral antioxidant treatment', *Human Reproduction*, Sep, 20(9), 2590–2594. Epub 2005 Jun 2.

[10] Bent, G. *et al*, 1993, `Folinic acid in the treatment of human male infertility', *Fertility and Sterility*, Oct, 60(4), 698–701.

[11] ASH, `Smoking and Reproduction', *Research studies fact sheet*, 2000.

[12] Munafo, M. *et al*, 2002, 'Does cigarette smoking increase time to conception?', *Journal of Biosocial Science*, 34, 65–73.

[13] Kinney, A. *et al*, 2007, `Smoking, alcohol and caffeine in relation to ovarian age during the reproductive years', *Human Reproduction*, Apr, 22(4), 1175–1185.

[14] Himmelberger, D.U. *et al*, 1998, `Cigarette smoking during pregnancy and the occurrence of spontaneous abortion and congenital abnormality', *American Journal of Epidemiology*, 108, 470–479.

[15] Meeker, J.D. *et al*, 2007, `Maternal exposure to second-hand tobacco smoke and pregnancy outcome among couples undergoing assisted reproduction', *Human Reproduction*, 22, 337–345.

[16] Mostafa, T. *et al*, 2006, `Effect of smoking on seminal plasma ascorbic acid in infertile and fertile males', *Andrologia*, 38, 221–224.

[17] Guo, H. *et al*, 2006, `Effects of cigarette, alcohol consumption and sauna on sperm morphology', *Zhonghua Nan Ke Xue*, 12, 215–217.

[18] Sorahan, T. *et al*, 1997, `Childhood cancer and parental use of tobacco: deaths from 1971 to 1976', *British Journal of Cancer*, 76, 1525–1531.

[19] Goldberg, C.A., 1999, `Cigarette after sex, or instead of it', *Muscular Development*, 36(3), 53.

[20] Sepaniak, S. *et al*, 2006, `Cigarette smoking and fertility in women and men', *Gynecology Obstetrique and Fertilite*, 34, 945–949.

[21] Klonoff-Cohen, H. *et al*, 2001, `Effects of female and male smoking on success rates of IVF and gamete intra-fallopian transfer', *Human Reproduction*, 16, 1382–1390.

[22] Linsten, A. *et al*, 2005, `Effects of subfertility cause, smoking and body weight on the success rate of IVF', *Human Reproduction*, Jul, 20(7), 1867–1875.

[23] Munafo, M. *et al*, 2002, 'Does cigarette smoking increase time to conception?', *Journal of Biosocial Science*, 34, 65–73.

[24] Li, Y. *et al*, 2005, `Maternal and grandmaternal smoking patterns are associated with early childhood asthma', *Chest*, Apr, 127(4), 1232–1241.

[25] Weinberg, C. *et al*, 1989, `Reduced fecundability in women with prenatal exposure to cigarette smoking', *American Journal of Epidemiology*, 129, 1972–1978; Golding, J., 1994, Royal Hospital for Children, Bristol, Talk given to a conference on Smoking in Pregnancy, commissioned by the Health Education Authority.

[26] Tuormaa, T. *et al*, 1995, `The adverse effects of tobacco smoking on reproduction and health: A review from the literature', *Nutrition and Health*, 10, 105–120.

[27] Goldberg, C., 1999, 'A cigarette after sex, or instead of it', *Muscular Development*, 36(3), 53.

[28] Tolstrup, J.S. *et al*, 2003, `Alcohol use as predictor for infertility in a representative population of Danish women', *Acta Obstetrics Gynecology Scandinavia*, 82, 744–749.

[29] Jensen, T.K. *et al*, 1998, 'Does moderate alcohol consumption affect fertility?', *British Medical Journal*, 317, 7157, 505–510.

[30] Eggert, J. *et al*, 2004, `Effects of alcohol consumption on female fertility during an 18 year period', *Fertility and Sterility*, 81, 379–383.

[31] Grodstein, F. *et al*, 1994, `Infertility in women and moderate alcohol use', *American Journal of Public Health*, 84, 1429–1432.

[32] Guo, H. *et al*, 2006, `Effects of cigarette, alcohol consumption and sauna on sperm morphology', *Zhonghua Nan Ke Xue*, 12, 215–217.

[33] Moran, L. *et al*, 2002, `The obese patient with infertility; a practical approach to diagnosis and treatment', *Nutrition in Clinical Care*, 5, p290–297.

[34] Holmes, T. *et al*, 1994, `Relations of exercise to body image and sexual desirability among a sample of university students', *Psychology Reports*, 74, 920–922.

[35] Hoeger, K. *et al*, 2007, `Obesity and lifestyle management in polycystic ovary syndrome', *Clinical Obstetrics and Gynecology*, Mar, 50(1), 277–294.

[36] Warren, M. *et al*, 2001, `The effects of intense exercise on the female reproductive system', *Journal of Endocrinology*, 170, 3–11.

[37] Spiegel, K. *et al*, 1999, `Impact of sleep on metabolic

and endocrine function', *Lancet*, 354, 1435–1439.

[38] Cutler, W. *et al*, 1985, `Sexual behaviour frequency and biphasic ovulatory type menstrual cycles', *Physiology Behaviour*, 34, 804–810; van Roijen, J. *et al*, 1996, `Sexual arousal and the quality of semen produced by masturbation', *Human Reproduction*, 11, 147–151.

[39] 'Orgasm wars', Jan/Feb 1996, *Psychology Today*.

[40] Cutler, W. *et al*, 1985, `Sexual behaviour frequency and biphasic ovulatory type menstrual cycles', *Physiology Behaviour*, 34, 804–810.

[41] *The initial investigation and management of the infertile couple: evidence based clinical guidelines*, no 2, Royal College of Obstetricians and Gynaeocologists (Feb 1998).

[42] Watanabe, G. *et al*, 1977, `Environmental determinants of birth defect prevalence', *Birth Defects Research Part A: Clinical and Molecular Teratology*, 16(3), 367.

[43] Kocisova, J. *et al*, 1988, `Mutagenicity studies on paracetamol in human volunteers: I Cytogenetic analysis of peripheral lymphocytes and lipid peroxidation in plasmas', *Mutation Research*, 209, 161–165.

[44] Stutz, G. *et al*, 2004, `The effect of alcohol, tobacco and aspirin consumption on seminal quality among healthy young men', *Archives of Environmental Health*, 59, 548–552.

[45] Reuhl, J. *et al*, 2001, `Morphometric assessment of testicular changes in drug-related fatalities', *Forensic Science International*, Jan, 15, 115(3), 171–178.

[46] Klonoff-Cohen, H. *et al*, 2001, `Maternal and paternal recreational drug use and sudden infant death syndrome', *Archives of Pediatrics and Adolescent Medicine*, July, 155, 7, 765–770.

[47] Powell, D. *et al*, 1983, `Marijuana and sex: strange bed partners', *Journal of Psychoactive Drugs*, 15, 169–280.

[48] Bracken, M. *et al*, 1999, `Association of cocaine use with sperm concentration, motility and morphology', *Fertility and Sterility*, 53, 315–322; Smith, C. *et al*, 1985, `Drug abuse effects on reproductive hormones', Thomas, J. *et al* (eds), *Endocrine Toxocology*, Raven Press, New York.

[49] Bongol, N. *et al*, 1987, `Teratogenicity of cocaine in humans', *Journal of Pediatrics*, 1, 93–96; Ostrea, E. *et al*, 1979, `Perinatal problems in maternal drug addiction: a study of 830 cases', *Journal of Pediatrics*, 94, 292–295.

[50] Stenchever, M. *et al*, 1974, `Chromosome breakages in users of marijuana', *American Journal of Obstetrics and Gynaecology*, 118, 106–113.

[51] Bongol, N. *et al*, 1987, `Teratogenicity of cocaine in humans', *Journal of Pediatrics*, 1, 93–96.

[52] Barena, E. *et al*, 1991, `Stress related reproductive failure', *Journal of IVF Embryo Transfer*, 8, 15–23.

[53] Maconochie, N. *et al*, 2007, `Risk factors for first trimester miscarriage – results from a UK-population-based case-control study', *British Journal of General Practice*, Feb, 114(2), 170–86; Jakobovits, A. *et al*, 2002, `Interactions of stress and reproduction', *Zentralblatt Gynakol*, 124, 189–193.

[54] Giblin, P. *et al*, 1988, `Effects of stress and characteristic adaptability on semen quality in healthy men', *Fertility and Sterility*, 49, 127–132.

[55] Lenzi, A. *et al*, 2003, `Stress, sexual dysfunctions and male infertility', *Journal of Endocrinological Investigation*, 26, 72–76.

[56] Fenster, L. *et al*, 'Effects of psychological stress on human semen quality', *Journal of Andrology*, 18, 2, 194–202.

[57] Clarke *et al*, 1999, `Relationship between psychological stress and semen quality among in-vitro fertilization patients', *Human Reproduction*, Mar, 14(3), 753–758.

[58] Vin, F. *et al*, 2007, `Effects of acute stress on the day of proestrus on sexual behaviour and ovulation in female rats: Participation of the angiotensinergic system', *Physiology and Behaviour*, May 22; Benedeck, T., 1939, 'Correlations between ovarian activity and psychodynamic processes. The annovulatory phase', *Psychosomatic Medicine*, 1(2), 245–270.

[59] Domar, A.D.R. *et al*, 1999, `Distress and conception in infertile women: A complementary approach', *Journal of the American Medical Women's Association*, 45, 4.

[60] Reiko, K. *et al*, 2002, `Work related reproductive disorders among working women', *Industrial Health*, 40, 101–112.

[61] Loftus, T. *et al*, 1962, `Psychogenic factors in anovulatory behaviour and psychoanalytic aspects of anovulatory amenorrhea', *Fertility and Sterility*, 13, 20; Cutler, W. *et al*, 1985, `Sexual behaviour frequency and biphasic ovulatory type menstrual

cycles', *Physiology and Behaviour,* 34, 805–810.

[62] Chang, R. *et al*, 2002, `Role of acupuncture in the treatment of female infertility', *Fertility and Sterility,* Dec, 78(6), 1149–1153; Johnston, D. *et al*, 2006, `Acupuncture prior to and at embryo transfer in an assisted conception unit – a case series', *Acupuncture in Medicine,* Mar, 24(1), 23–28; West, L. *et al*, 2006, `Acupuncture on the day of embryo transfer significantly improves reproductive outcome in infertile women: a prospective, randomized trial', *Fertility and Sterility,* May, 85(5), 1341–1346. Epub 2006 Apr 5.

[63] Diet, S. *et al*, 2006, `Effect of acupuncture on the outcome of in vitro fertilization and intracytoplasmic sperm injection: a randomized, prospective, controlled clinical study', *Fertility and Sterility,* May, 85(5), 1347–1351. Epub 2006 Apr 17; Yang, J. *et al*, 2005, `Controlled study on acupuncture for treatment of endocrine dysfunctional infertility', *Zhongguo Zhen Jiu,* May, 25(5), 299–300; Chen, B.Y. *et al*, 1997, `Acupuncture normalises dysfunction of hypothalmic-pituitary ovarian axis', *Acupuncture Electrotherapy Research,* 22 (2), 97–108; Stener-Victorin, E. *et al*, 2000, `Effects of electro-acupuncture on anovulation in women with polycystic ovary syndrome', *Acta Obstetrics Gynecology Scandinavia,* Mar, 79(3), 180–188; Liao, D.L. *et al*, 1989, `Influence of artificial cycles induced by traditional Chinese medicine on the releasing and reserving gonadotrophic hormone function of the pituitary gland in the female with secondary amenorrhea', *Zhong Xi Yi Jie He Za Zhi,* Aug 9(8), 458–461.

[64] Beal, M. *et al*, 1998, `Women's use of complementary and alternative therapies in reproductive health care', *Journal of Nurse-Midwifery,* May–Jun, 43(3), 224–34.

[65] Gerhar, I. *et al*, 2002, `Individualized homeopathic therapy for male infertility', *Homeopathy,* Jul, 91(3), 133–44.

[66] Association of Relexologists, *http://www.aor.org.uk/index.asp?page=research*

[67] Erikson, Leila, Chairman of the Forenede Danske Zneterapeuter (Danish Reflexology Association) Research Committee, 1994, `Has reflexology an effect on fertility?'

[68] Chigbugh, A., 1975, `Psychomatic sterility and psychosomatic infertility', *Rivista Internazionale di Psicologia e Ipnosi,* Jan–Mar 16, 91, 37–41.

[69] Mikesell, S.G., 2000, `Infertility and pregnancy loss – hypnotic interventions for reproductive challenges', in Horbyak, L.M. *et al*, (eds), *Healing from within: the use of hypnosis in women's health care,* The American Psychological Association, Washington DC.

[70] Muzz, L. *et al*, 2006, `Aromatherapy and reducing preprocedural anxiety: A controlled prospective study', *Gastroenterology Nursing,* Nov–Dec, 29(6), 466–471; Perry, N. *et al*, 2006, `Aromatherapy in the management of psychiatric disorders: clinical and neuropharmacological perspectives', *CNS Drugs,* 20(4) 257–280.

STEP THREE
FERTILITY-BOOSTING SUPPLEMENTS

[1] Gill, I. *et al*, 2006, `Quality changes and nutrient retention in fresh-cut versus whole fruits during storage', *Journal of Agricultural Food Chemistry,* Jun 14, 54(12), 4284–4296; Reddy, M. *et al*, 1999, `The impact of food processing on the nutritional quality of vitamins and minerals', *Advanced Experimental Medicine and Biology,* 459, 99–106.

[2] Shroeder, H. *et al*, 1971, `Losses of vitamins and trace minerals resulting from processing and preservation of foods', *American Journal of Clinical Nutrition,* May, 24(5), 562–573.

[3] Ebisch, I. *et al*, 2007, `The importance of folate, zinc and antioxidants in the pathogenesis and prevention of subfertility', *Human Reproduction Update,* Mar–Apr, 13(2), 163–174. Epub 2006 Nov 11.

[4] Forges, T., 2007, `Impact of folate and homocysteine metabolism on human reproductive health', *Human Reproduction Update,* May–Jun, 13(3), 225–238. Epub 2007 Feb 16; Czeizel, A. *et al*, 1998, `Periconceptional folic acid containing multivitamin supplementation', *European Journal of Obstetrical Gynecological Reproductive Biology,* Jun, 78(2), 151–161.

[5] Ebisch, I. *et al*, 2006, `Does folic acid and zinc sulphate intervention affect endocrine parameters and sperm characteristics in men?', *International Journal of Andrology,* Apr, 29(2), 339–345.

[6] Schwabe, J. *et al*, 1991, `Beyond zinc fingers', *Trends in Biochemical Sciences* 16, 291–296.

[7] Hurley, L. *et al*, 1991, `Teratogenic aspects of

manganese, zinc and copper nutrition', *Physiological Reviews*, 61, 249–295.

[8] Lin, Y.C., 2000, `Seminal plasma zinc levels and sperm motion characteristics in infertile samples', *Changgeng Yi Xue Za Zhi*, May, 23(5), 260–266; Hunt, D. *et al*, 1992, `Effects of dietary zinc depletion on seminal volume and zinc loss, serum concentration and sperm morphology in young men,' *American Journal of Clinical Nutrition* 56, 148–157.

[9] Hunt, D. *et al*, 1992, `Effects of dietary zinc depletion', *American Journal of Clinical Nutrition*, 56, 150–154.

[10] Al Kunani, A. *et al*, 2001, `The selenium status of women with a history of recurrent miscarriage', *British Journal of General Practice*, Oct, 108(10), 1094–1097.

[11] Kestes, A., 2003, `Sperm oxidative stress and the effect of an oral vitamin E and selenium supplement on semen quality in infertile men', *Archives of Andrology*, Mar–Apr, 49(2), 83–94.

[12] Krxnjavi, H. *et al*, 1992, `Selenium and fertility in men', *Trace Elements in Medicine*, 9, 2, 107–108; Scott, R. *et al*, 1997, `Selenium supplementation in subfertile human males', in Fischer , P.W.F. *et al*, *Trace Elements in Man and Animals*, Ottawa: NCR Research Press 9; Scott, R., 1998, `The effect of oral selenium supplementation on human sperm motility', *British Journal of Urology*, 82, 76–80.

[13] Geva, E. *et al*, 1996, `The effect of anti-oxidant treatment on human spermatozoa and fertilization rate in an in vitro fertilization programme', *Fertility and Sterility*, 66(3), 430–434; Kestes, A.L. *et al*, 2003, `Sperm oxidative stress and the effect of an oral vitamin E and selenium supplement on semen quality in infertile men', *Archives of Andrology*, Mar–Apr, 49(2), 83–94; Koca, Y., 2003, `Antioxidant activity of seminal plasma in fertile and infertile men', *Archives of Andrology*, Sep–Oct, 49(5), 355–359.

[14] Simopoulos, A.O., 1991, `Omega 3 fatty acids in health and disease and in growth and development', *American Journal of Clinical Nutrition*, 54, 438–463.

[15] McGregor, G. *et al*, 2001, `The omega-3 story: nutritional prevention of preterm birth and other adverse pregnancy outcomes', *Obstetrical and Gynecological Survey*, May, 56(5 Suppl 1), S1–13.

[16] Rossi, E. *et al*, 1993, `Fish oil derivatives as a prophylaxis of recurrent miscarriage associated with antiphospholipid antibodies (APL): a pilot study', *Lupus*, Oct, 2(5), 319–323; Prescott, E. *et al*, 2007, `Maternal fish oil supplementation in pregnancy modifies neonatal leukotriene production by cord blood derived neutrophils', *Clinical Science (London)*, Jun 28.

[17] Aksoy, Y. *et al*, 2006, `Sperm fatty acid composition in subfertile men', *Prostaglandins Leukotrienes and Essential Fatty Acids*, Aug, 75(2), 75–79.

[18] Ronnen, A. *et al*, 2007, `Preconception B-Vitamin and Homocysteine Status, Conception, and Early Pregnancy Loss', *American Journal of Epidemiology*, May 2; Bendich, A. *et al*, 2000, `The potential for dietary supplements to reduce premenstrual syndrome (PMS) symptoms', *Journal of the American College of Nutrition*, Feb, 19(1), 3–12; Kidd, D. *et al*, 1982, `The effects of pyridoxine on pituitary hormone secretion in amenorrhea-galactorrhea syndromes', *Journal of Clinical Endocrinology and Metabolism*, Apr, 54(4), 872–875.

[19] Kidd, G. *et al*, 1982, `The effects of pyridoxine on pituitary hormone secretion in amenorrhea', *Journal of Clinical Endocrinology and Metabolism*, 54, 872–875.

[20] Beenet, M., 2001, `Vitamin B12 deficiency, infertility and recurrent fetal loss', *Journal of Reproductive Medicine*, (01)Mar, 46(3), 209–212.

[21] Bayer R., 1960, `Treatment of infertility with vitamin E', *International Journal of Fertility*, 5, 70–78.

[22] Tarin, J. *et al*, 1998, `Effects of maternal ageing and dietary antioxidant supplementation on ovulation, fertilisation and embryo development in vitro in the mouse', *Reproduction, Nutrition, Development*, Sep–Oct, 38(5), 499–508; Bates, C.J., 2002, `Plasma carotenoid and vitamin E concentrations in women living in a rural west African (Gambian) community', *International Journal of Vitamin and Nutrition Research*, May, 72(3), 133–141.

[23] Kestes, A.L. *et al*, 2003, `Sperm oxidative stress and the effect of an oral vitamin e and selenium supplement on semen quality in infertile men', *Archives of Andrology*, Mar–Apr, 49(2), 83–94; Koca, Y., 2003, `Antioxidant activity of seminal plasma in fertile and infertile men', *Archives of Andrology*, Sep–Oct, 49(5), 355–359.

[24] Geva, E. *et al*, 1996, `The effect of anti-oxidant treatment on human spermatozoa and fertilization

rate in an in vitro fertilization programme', *Fertility and Sterility* 66, 3, 430–434.

[25] Acuff, A. *et al*, 1998, `Transport of deuterium-labeled tocopherols during pregnancy', *American Journal of Clinical Nutrition*, Mar, 67(3), 459–464.

[26] Crha, I., 2003, `Ascorbic acid and infertility treatment', *Central European Journal of Public Health*, Jun, 11(2), 63–67.

[27] Fraga, C. *et al*, 1991, `Ascorbic acid protects against endogenous oxidative DNA damage in human sperm', *Proceedings of the National Academy of Science* 88, 11003–11006; Dawson, E.B. *et al*, 1987, `Effect of ascorbic acid on male fertility', *Annuals of New York Academy of Science,* 498, 812–828.

[28] Mostafa, T. *et al*, 2006, `Effect of smoking on seminal plasma ascorbic acid in infertile and fertile males', *Andrologia,* 38, 221–224.

[29] Song, G. *et al*, 2006, `Relationship between seminal ascorbic acid and sperm DNA integrity in infertile men', *International Journal of Andrology*, Dec, 29(6), 569–575.

[30] Chavarro, J. *et al*, 2006, `Iron intake and risk of ovulatory infertility', *Obstetrics and Gynecology*, Nov, 108(5), 1145–1152.

[31] Zdziennicki, A., 1996, `Iron deficiency as a risk factor during the perinatal period', *Ginekologia Polska*, Jun, 67(6), 301–303.

[32] Morales, M. *et al*, 2003, `Progressive motility increase caused by L-arginine and polyamines in sperm from patients with idiopathic and diabetic asthenozoospermia', *Ginecologia y Obstetricia de Mexico*, Jun, 71, 297–303; Bridge, C. *et al*, 1998, `The administration of L-arginine to enhance male fertility' (Dissertation for the *Institute of Optimum Nutrition* Diploma Course); de Aloysio, D. *et al*, 1982, `The clinical use of arginine asparate in male infertility', *Acta Europaea Fertilitatis,* 13, 133–167.

[33] Battaglia, C. *et al*, 1999, `Adjuvant L-arginine treatment for in-vitro fertilization in poor responder patients', *Human Reproduction,* 14, 1690–1697.

[34] Vitali, G. *et al*, 1995, `Carnitine supplementation in human idiopathic asthenospermia', *Drugs under Experimental and Clinical Research,* 21, 157–168; Lenzi, A., 2003, `Use of carnitine therapy in selected cases of male factor infertility: a double-blind crossover trial', *Fertility and Sterility*, Feb, 79(2), 292–300.

[35] Balercia, G. *et al*, 2002, `Coenzyme Q10 levels in idiopathic and varicocele-associated asthenozoospermia', *Andrologia,* 34(2),107–111.

[36] Balercia, G. *et al*, 2004, `Coenzyme Q(10) supplementation in infertile men with idiopathic asthenozoospermia: an open, uncontrolled pilot study', *Fertility and Sterility,* 81(1), 93–98.

[37] Katz, J. *et al*, 2000, `Maternal low-dose vitamin A or beta-carotene supplementation has no effect on fetal loss and early infant mortality: a randomized cluster trial in Nepal', *American Journal of Clinical Nutrition*, Jun, 71(6), 1570–1576.

[38] Cahill, D.J. *et al*, 1994, `Multiple follicular development associated with herbal medicine', *Human Reproduction (UK)* 9(8), 1469–1470.

[39] Propping, D. *et al*, 1987, `Treatment of corpus luteum insufficiency', *Zeitschr Allgemainmedizin* 63, 932–933; Sliutz, G. *et al*, 1993, `Agnus Castus extract inhibits prolactin secretion of rat pituitary cells', *Hormone and Metabolic Research* 25, 253–255; Jarry, H. *et al*, 1994, `In vitro prolactin but not LH and FSH release is inhibited by compounds in extracts of Agnus castus: direct evidence for a dopaminergic principle by the dopamine receptor assay', *Experimental and Clinical Endocrinology,* 102(6), 448–454.

[40] Chaing, H. *et al*, 1994, `Medicinal plants: Conception/contraception', *Advanced Contraceptive Delivery Systems.,* 10, 3–4. 355–363.

[41] Sikora, R. *et al*, 1989, `Ginkgo biloba extract in the therapy of erectile dysfunction', *Journal of Urology,* 141, 188A.

[42] Kim, D.H., 2003, `Effects of ginseng saponin on hypothalamo-pituitary-adrenal axis in mice', *Neuroscience Letter,* 343, 62–66.

[43] Czeizel, A., 1996, `The effect of preconceptional multivitamin supplementation on fertility', *International Journal of Vitamin and Nutrition Research,* 66, 55–58; Glenville, M. *et al*, 2006, `Nutritional supplements in pregnancy: commercial push or evidence based?', *Current Opinion in Obstetrics and Gynecology*, Dec, 18(6), 642–647.

STEP FOUR
ELIMINATE ENVIRONMENTAL AND OCCUPATIONAL HAZARDS

[1] 'Chemicals and Health' – *www.foe.co.uk*

[2] Baranski, B., 1993, `Effects of workplace on fertility

and related reproductive outcome', *Environmental Health Perspectives*, 101, 2, Suppl., 81–90.

3 Sirakov, M. *et al*, 2004, `Xenoestrogens – danger for the future generations?', *Akush Ginekol (Sofiia)*, 43(4), 39–45.

4 Singleton, D. *et al*, 2003, `Xenoestrogen exposure and mechanisms of endocrine disruption', *Frontiers in Bioscience*, Jan 1, 8, s110–118.

5 Sharpe, R.M. *et al*, 2002, `Environment, lifestyle and infertility – an inter-generational issue', *Nature Cell Biology*, Oct, 4 Suppl, s33–40.

6 Ropstad, F. *et al*, 2006, `Endocrine Disruption Induced by Organochlorines (OCs): Field Studies And Experimental Models', *Journal of Toxicology and Environmental Health A*, Jan, 69(1), 53–76; 2001, Ibareta, D. *et al*, 'Possible health impact of phytoestrogens and xenoestrogens in food', *Acta Pathologica Microbiologica et Immunologica Scandinavia*, Mar, 109(3), 161–184.

7 Bretveld, R.W. *et al*, 2006, `Pesticide exposure: the hormonal function of the female reproductive system disrupted?', *Reproductive Biology and Endocrinology*, May 31, 4, 30.

8 Meeker, J.D. *et al*, 2006, `Exposure to nonpersistent insecticides and male reproductive hormones', *Epidemiology*, 17, 61–68.

9 Sug, O. *et al*, 2005, `Exposure to bisphenol A is associated with recurrent miscarriage', *Human Reproduction*, Aug, 20(8), 2325–2329. Epub 2005 Jun 9. *Human Reproduction Journal*, June 2005.

10 Ohash, A. *et al*, 2005, `Evaluation of endocrine disrupting activity of plasticizers in polyvinyl chloride tubes by estrogen receptor alpha binding assay', *Journal of Artificial Organs*, 8(4), 252–256.

11 Nuti, F. *et al*, 2005, `Synthesis of DEHP metabolites as biomarkers for GC-MS evaluation of phthalates as endocrine disrupters', *Bioorganic and Medicinal Chemistry*, May 16, 13(10), 3461–3465.

12 Katsu, Y. *et al*, 2007, `Functional associations between two estrogen receptors, environmental estrogens, and sexual disruption in the roach (Rutilus rutilus)', *Environmental Science and Technology*, May 1, 41(9), 3368–3374.

13 http://news.bbc.co.uk/1/hi/health/3545684.stm; http://www.dwi.gov.uk/pressrel/2004/pr0304.shtm

14 Baranski, B., 1993, `Effects of workplace on fertility and related reproductive outcome', *Environmental Health Perspectives Supplements*, 101, (2, Suppl.), 81–90.

15 Winder, C. *et al*, 1993, `Lead, reproduction and development', *Neurotoxicology*, 14, 303; Tabacova S. *et al*, 1993, *Environmental Health Perspectives Supplements*, 101(2), 27–31; Bogden, J.D. *et al*, 1997, `Lead poisoning – one approach to a problem that won't go away', *Environmental Health Perspectives*, 105(12), 1284–1287; Coste J. *et al*, 1991, 'Lead-exposed workmen and fertility: A study of 354 subjects', *European Journal of Epidemiology*, 7, 154–158; Chuang, H. *et al*, 2005, `Estimation of burden of lead for offspring of female lead workers: a quality-adjusted life year (QALY) assessment', *Journal of Toxicology and Environmental Health*, Sep, 68(17–18), 1485–1496; Maizlish, N. *et al*, 1988, `Mortality among California highway workers', *American Journal of Industrial Medicine*, 13(3), 363–379.

16 Myl, A. *et al*, 2004, `Inhibitory effect of cadmium and tobacco alkaloids on expansion of porcine oocyte-cumulus complexes', *Central European Journal of Public Health*, Mar, 12 Suppl, S62–64; Beoff, S. *et al*, 2000, `Male infertility and environmental exposure to lead and cadmium', *Human Reproduction Update*, Mar–Apr, 6(2), 107–121; Ward, N. *et al*, 1987, `Placental element levels in relation to foetal development of obstetrically normal births: A study of 39 elements. Evidence for effects of cadmium, lead and zinc on foetal growth', *International Journal of Biosocial Research*, 9(1).

17 Giudice, L. *et al*, 2006, `Infertility and the environment: the medical context', *Seminars in Reproductive Medicine*, Jul, 24(3), 129–133; Gerhard, I. *et al*, 1998, `Heavy metals and fertility', *Journal of Toxicology and Environmental Health*, 54(8), 593–611.

18 Choy, C.M. *et al*, 2002, `Infertility, blood mercury concentrations and dietary seafood consumption: a case-control study', *British Journal of General Practice*, Oct, 109(10), 1121–1125; Weber, R.F. *et al*, 2000, `Male fertility. Possibly affected by occupational exposure to mercury', *Nederlands Tijdschrift voor Tandheelkunde*, Dec, 107(12), 495–498; Davies, B.J. *et al*, 2001, `Mercury vapor and female reproductive toxicity', *Toxicological Science*, Feb, 59(2), 291–296; Moszczynski, P. *et al*, 1997, `P Mercury compounds and the immune system: A review', *International Journal of Occupational Medicine and Environmental*

Health, 10(3), 247–258; Castoldi, A., 2003, `Neurotoxic and molecular effects of ethylmercury in humans', *Reviews on Environmental Health,* Jan–Mar, 18(1), 19–31.

[19] Olfert, S. *et al,* 2006, `Reproductive outcomes among dental personnel: a review of selected exposures', *Journal of Canadian Dental Association,* Nov, 72(9), 821–825; Rowland, A.S. *et al,* 1994, `The effect of occupational exposure to mercury vapour on the fertility of female dentists', *Occupational and Environmental Medicine* 51, 1, 28–34.

[20] Gerahard, I. *et al,* 1991, `Unexplained infertility in women with high levels of decorating/furnishing chemicals: prolonged exposure to wood preservatives causes endocrine and immunological disorders in women', *American Journal of Obstetrics and Gynecology,* 165, 92.

[21] Kaniwa, A. *et al,* 2006, `Preventive measures against health damage due to chemicals in household products', *Kokuritsu Iyakuhin Shokuh,* 124, 1–20.

[22] Axmon, A. *et al,* 2006, `Fertility among female hairdressers', *Scandinavian Journal of Work, Environment and Health,* Feb, 32(1), 51–60.

[23] Karp, J. *et al,* 2006, `Health risk assessment of occupational exposure to a magnetic field from magnetic resonance imaging devices', *International Journal of Occupational Safety and Ergonomics,* 12(2), 155–167; WHO's health risk assessment of ELF fields, 2003, *Radiation Protection Dosimetry,* 106(4), 297–299.

[24] Agarwal, A. *et al,* 2007, `Effect of cell phone usage on semen analysis in men attending infertility clinic: an observational study', *Fertility and Sterility,* May 3.

[25] Rig, A. *et al,* 2007, `Dietary exposure to methyl mercury and PCB and the associations with semen parameters among Swedish fishermen', *Environmental Health,* May 8, 6.

[26] Schrumpf, A. *et al,* 1975, `Texture of broccoli and carrots cooked by microwave energy', *Journal of Food Science,* 40, 1025–1029.

[27] Maureen, P. *et al,* 1997, `Occupational reproductive hazards', *Lancet,* 349, 1385–1388.

[28] McDiarmid, M. *et al,* 2006, `Preconception brief: occupational/environmental exposures', *Maternal and Child Health Journal,* Sep, 10(5 Suppl), S123–128. Epub 2006 Aug 8; Figa-Talamanca, I. *et al,* 2006, `Occupational risk factors and reproductive health of women', *Occupational Medicine (London),* Dec, 56(8), 521–531; Figa-Talamanca, I., 2001, `Occupational exposures to metals, solvents and pesticides: recent evidence on male reproductive effects and biological markers', *Occupational Medicine (London),* 51(3), 174–188.

[29] Figa, I. *et al,* 1996, `Effects of prolonged autovehicle driving on male reproduction function: a study among taxi drivers', *American Journal of Industrial Medicine,* Dec, 30(6), 750–758.

[30] Figa, I. *et al,* 1992, `Fertility and semen quality of workers exposed to high temperatures in the ceramics industry', *Reproductive Toxicology,* 6(6), 517–523.

[31] Sallmen, M. *et al,* 2006, `Fertility and exposure to solvents among families in the Agricultural Health Study', *Occupational and Environmental Medicine,* Jul, 63(7), 469–475. Epub 2006 May 12.

[32] Yucra, S. *et al,* 2006, `Semen quality and reproductive sex hormone levels in Peruvian pesticide sprayers', *International Journal of Occupational and Environmental Health,* Oct–Dec, 12(4), 355–361.

[33] Ahlborg, J. *et al,* 1995, `Reproductive effects of chemical exposures in health professions', *Journal of Occupational and Environmental Medicine,* 37; Claman, P. *et al,* 2004, `Men at risk: occupation and male infertility', *Fertility and Sterility,* Mar, 81, Suppl 2, 19–26.

[34] Kenkel, S. *et al,* 2001, `Occupational risks for male fertility: an analysis of patients attending a tertiary referral centre', *International Journal of Andrology,* Dec, 24(6), 318–326.

[35] Chen, P. *et al,* 2002, `Prolonged time to pregnancy in female workers exposed to ethylene glycol ethers in semiconductor manufacturing', *Epidemiology,* Mar, 13(2), 191–196; Multingner, L. *et al,* 2007, `Glycol ethers and semen quality: a cross-sectional study among male workers in the Paris Municipality', *Occupational and Environmental Medicine,* Jul, 64(7), 467–473. Epub 2007 Mar 1.

[36] Abell, A. *et al,* 2000, `Time to pregnancy among female greenhouse workers', *Scandinavian Journal of Work, Environment and Health,* Apr, 26(2), 131–136; Sinawat, S. *et al,* 2000, `The environmental impact on male fertility', *Journal of Medicine Association of Thailand,* Aug, 83(8), 880–885.

[37] Laslo-Baker, D. *et al*, 2004, `Child neurodevelopmental outcome and maternal occupation exposure to solvents', *Archives of Pediatrics and Adolescent Medicine*, 158, 956–961.

[38] Bar, P. *et al*, 2006, `The effect of women's occupational psychologic stress on outcome of fertility treatments', *Journal of Occupational and Environmental Medicine*, Jan, 48(1), 56–62.

[39] Zhl, J. *et al*, 2003, `Shift work and subfecundity: a causal link or an artefact?', *Journal of Occupational and Environmental Medicine*, Sep, 60(9), E12; Ahlborg, G. *et al*, 1996, `Shift work, nitrous oxide exposure and subfertility among Swedish midwives', *International Journal of Epidemiology*, Aug, 25(4), 783–790.

[40] Gracia, C. *et al*, 2005, `Occupational exposures and male infertility', *American Journal of Epidemiology*, Oct 15, 162(8), 729–733. Epub 2005 Aug 24.

[41] Tunt, P. *et al*, 1998, `Are long working hours and shift work risk factors for subfecundity? A study among couples from southern Thailand', *Journal of Occupational and Environmental Medicine*, Feb, 55(2), 99–105; Feinberg, J. *et al*, 1998, `Pregnant workers. A physician's guide to assessing safe employment', *Western Journal of Medicine*, Feb, 168(2), 86–92; Chia, S. *et al*, 1994, `Study of the effects of occupation and industry on sperm quality', *Annuals, Academy of Medicine Singapore*, Sep, 23(5), 645–649.

[42] Goldhaber, M. *et al*, 1988, `The risk of miscarriage and birth defects among women who use VDUs during pregnancy', *American Journal of Industrial Medicine*, 13, 695–706.

[43] `Japanese miscarriages blamed on computer terminals', 1985, *New Scientist*, 23 May.

[44] Sheynkin, Y. *et al*, 2005, `Increase in scrotal temperature in laptop computer users', *Human Reproduction*, Feb, 20(2), 452–455. Epub 2004 Dec 9.

STEP FIVE
SCREENING FOR INFECTIONS

[1] Gomez, C. *et al*, 1979, `Attachment of Neisseria gonorrhoea to human sperm', *British Journal of Venereal Disease*, 55, 245–255.

[2] Pavletic, A. *et al*, 1999, `Infertility following pelvic inflammatory disease', *Infectious Diseases in Obstetrics and Gynecology*, 7(3), 145–152; Westroom, L. *et al*, 1995, `Effect of pelvic inflammatory disease on fertility', *Venereology*, Nov, 8(4), 219–222.

[3] Royal College of Physicians Committee on GU Medicine, 1987, `Chlamydia diagnostic services in the UK and Eire: current facilities and perceived needs', *Genitourinary Medicine*, 62, 371–374.

[4] Maeda, S. *et al*, 2007, `Treatment of men with urethritis negative for Neisseria gonorrhoea, Chlamydia trachomatis, Mycoplasma genitalium, Mycoplasma hominis, Ureaplasma parvum and Ureaplasma urealyticum', *International Journal of Urology*, May, 14(5), 422–425.

[5] Andrews, W.W. *et al*, 2000, `The preterm prediction study: association of second-trimester genitourinary Chlamydia infection with subsequent spontaneous preterm birth', *American Journal of Obstetrics and Gynecology*, 183, 3, Sep, 662–668.

[6] Kalwij, S. *et al*, 2007, `Time for action on Chlamydia', *British Medical Journal*, Apr 21, 334(7598), 813.

[7] Bar, N. *et al*, 1993, `Infection and pyospermia in male infertility', *World Journal of Urology*, 11(2), 76–81; Centre for Disease Control and Prevention, 2000–2005, `Increases in gonorrhea – eight western states', *Morbidity and Mortality Weekly Report*, 2007, Mar 16, 56(10), 222–225.

[8] Morency, A. *et al*, 2007, `The effect of second-trimester antibiotic therapy on the rate of preterm birth', *Journal of Obstetrics and Gynaecology Canada*, Jan, 29(1), 35–44.

[9] Klebanoff, S. *et al*, 1991, `Control of the microbial flora of the vagina by H2O2-generating lactobacilli', *Journal of Infectious Diseases*, 164, 94–100.

[10] Cotch, M. *et al*, 1997, `Trichomonas vaginalis associated with low birth weight and preterm delivery. The Vaginal Infections and Prematurity Study Group', *Sexually Transmitted Diseases*, Jul, 24(6), 353–360.

[11] Locksmith, G. *et al*, 2001, `Infection, antibiotics, and preterm delivery', *Seminars in Perinatology*, Oct, 25(5), 295–309.

[12] Tanaka, K. *et al*, 2006, `Screening for vaginal shedding of cytomegalovirus in healthy pregnant women using real-time PCR: correlation of CMV in the vagina and adverse outcome of pregnancy', *Journal of Medical Virology*, Jun, 78(6), 757–759.

[13] Kap, N. *et al*, 2003, `Detection of herpes simplex virus, cytomegalovirus, and Epstein-Barr virus in the semen of men attending an infertility clinic',

Fertility and Sterility, Jun, 79 Suppl 3, 1566–1570.

[14]Weidner, W. *et al*, 1985, `Ureaplasmal infections of the male urogenital tract, in particular prostatitis, and semen quality', *Urologia Internationlis*, 40(1), 5–9; Rose, B. *et al*, 1994, `Sperm motility, morphology, hyperactivation, and ionophore-induced acrosome reactions after overnight incubation with mycoplasmas', *Fertility and Sterility*, Feb, 61(2), 341–348.

[15] Clausen, H. *et al*, 2001, `Serological investigation of Mycoplasma genitalium in infertile women', *Human Reproduction*, Sep, 16(9), 1866–1874; Ye, E. *et al*, 2004, `Relationship between the endocervical mycoplasma infection and spontaneous abortion due to early embryonic death', *Zhonghua Fu Chan Ke Za Zhi*, Feb, 39(2), 83–85.

[16]Benn, C. *et al*, 2002, `Maternal vaginal microflora during pregnancy and the risk of asthma hospitalization and use of antiasthma medication in early childhood', *Journal of Allergy and Clinical Immunology*, Jul, 110(1),72–77.

[17]Spin, A. *et al*, 1995, `The impact of oral contraception on vulvovaginal candidiasis', *Contraception*, May, 51(5), 293–297.

[18] Sulak, P. *et al*, 2003, `Sexually transmitted diseases', *Seminars in Reproductive Medicine*, Nov, 21(4), 399–413.

[19] Zhang, R. *et al*, 2006, `An intervention study on preventing maternal-fetal transmission of syphilis during pregnancy', *Zhonghua Liu Xing Bing Xue Za Zhi*, Oct, 27(10), 901–904.

[20] Gardella, C. *et al*, 2007, `Managing genital herpes infections in pregnancy', *Cleveland Clinic Journal of Medicine*, Mar, 74(3), 217–224.

[21] Silver, H. *et al*, 1998, `Listeriosis during pregnancy', *Obstetrical and Gynecological Survey*, Dec, 53(12), 737–740.

[22] Freud, V. *et al*, 1980, `Haemolytic streptococci of the serological group B and pneumococci – new life-threatening bacteria in newborn wards (author's transl)', *Zeitschrift fur Geburtshilfe und Perinatologie*, Apr, 184(2), 142–149.

STEP SIX
GETTING THE TIMING RIGHT

[1] Branigan, E.F. *et al*, 2003, `A randomized clinical trial of treatment of clomiphene citrate-resistant anovulation with the use of oral contraceptive pill suppression and repeat clomiphene citrate treatment', *American Journal of Obstetrics and Gynecology*, Jun, 188(6), 1424–1428.

[2] Spria, N., 1985, `Fertility of couples following cessation of contraception', *Journal of Biosocial Science*, Jul, 17(3), 281–290; Weisberg, E. *et al*, 1982, `Fertility after discontinuation of oral contraceptives', *Clinical Reproduction and Fertility*, Dec, 1(4), 261–272; Chasan-Tabar, L. *et al*, 1997, `Oral contraceptives and ovulatory causes of delayed fertility', *American Journal of Epidemiology*, Aug 1, 146(3), 258–265.

[3] La Vecchia, C. *et al*, 2006, `Oral contraceptives and cancer', *Minerva Ginecologica*, Jun, 58(3), 209–214.

[4] Tyrer, L.B. *et al*, 1984, `Nutrition and the pill', *Journal of Reproductive Medicine*, Jul, 547–550; and according to the *British Medical Association Official Guide to Medicines and Drugs*, Dorling Kindersley, 1998, 147.

[5] Philips, O. *et al*, 2001, `New aspects of injectable contraception', *International Journal of Fertility and Women's Medicine*, Jan–Feb, 46(1), 31–36.

[6] Rivera, R. and Rountree, W., 2003, `Characteristics of menstrual problems associated with Norplant discontinuation: results of a multinational study', *Contraception*, 67(5), 373–377.

[7] Perloff, W., 1964, `In vitro survival of spermatozoa in cervical mucous', *American Journal of Obstetrics and Gynecology*, 88, 439–442.

[8] Baerwald, A.R. *et al*, 2003, 'A new model for ovarian follicular development during the human menstrual cycle', *Fertility and Sterility*, 80, 1, 116–122.

[9] Cutler, W.B. *et al*, 1985, `Sexual behaviour frequency and biphasic ovulatory type menstrual cycles', *Physiology and Behaviour*, May, 34(5), 805–810.

[10]Levitas, E. *et al*, 2005, `Relationship between the duration of sexual abstinence and semen quality: analysis of 9,489 semen samples', *Fertility and Sterility*, Jun, 83(6), 1680–1686.

[11]Cossom, J. *et al*, 2003, `How spermatozoa come to be confined to surfaces', *Cell Motility and the Cytoskeleton*, Jan, 54(1), 56–63.

STEP SEVEN FERTILITY TESTS

[1] Soules, M.R., *et al*, 2001, `Executive summary: Stages of Reproductive Aging Workshop (STRAW)', *Fertility and Sterility*, 5, 874–878.

[2] Abdalla, H. and Thum, M.Y., 2004, `An elevated

basal FSH reflects a quantitative rather than qualitative decline of the ovarian reserve', *Human Reproduction,* 19, 893–898.

3 Van Rooij, I.J., 2003, `Women older than 40 years of age and those with elevated FSH hormone levels differ in poor response rate and embryo quality in in-vitro fertilization', *Fertility and Sterility,* 79, 482–488.

4 Sharif, K. and Afnan, K., 2003, `The IVF league tables: time for a reality check', *Human Reproduction,* 18, 484–485.

5 Guid Oei, S. *et al,* 1998, `Effectiveness of the post-coital test: randomised controlled trial', *British Medical Journal,* 317, 502–505.

6 Kud, A. *et al,* 2005, `Prediction of laparoscopic surgery outcomes in tubal infertility', *Australian and New Zealand Journal of Obstetrics and Gynaecology,* Oct, 45(5), 460–463.

7 Pires, E. *et al,* 2007, `Specific and Sensitive Immunoassays Detect Multiple Anti-ovarian Antibodies in Women With Infertility', *Journal of Histochemistry amd Cytochemistry,* 1181–1190; Stem, C. *et al,* 2006, `Antiphospholipid antibodies and coagulation defects in women with implantation failure after IVF and recurrent miscarriage', *Reproductive BioMedicine Online,* Jul, 13(1), 29–37.

8 Swan, S. *et al,* 2000, `The question of declining sperm density revisited: an analysis of 101 studies published 1934–1996', *Environmental Health Perspectives,* Oct, 108(10), 961–966; Golden, A. *et al,* 1999, `Male reproduction and environmental and occupational exposures: a review of epidemiologic methods', *Salud Publica de Mexico,* 41 Suppl 2, S93–105.

9 Hauser, H. *et al,* 2002, `Environmental organochlorines and semen quality: results of a pilot study', *Environmental Health Perspectives,* Mar, 110(3), 229–233.

10 Zorn, B. *et al,* 2007, `Psychological factors in male partners of infertile couples: relationship with semen quality and early miscarriage', *International Journal of Andrology,* Jul 25.

11 Ezeh, U.E. *et al,* 1998, `Correlation of testicular sperm extraction with morphological, biophysical and endocrine profiles in men with azoospermia due to primary gonadal failure', *Human Reproduction,* 13, 3066–3074.

12 Shamaly, H. *et al,* 2004, `Infertility and coeliac disease: do we need more than one serological marker?', *Acta Obstetrics and Gynecology Scandinavia,* Dec, 83(12), 1184–1188.

13 Goddard, C. *et al,* 2006, `Complications of coeliac disease: are all patients at risk?', *Postgraduate Medical Jounal,* Nov, 82(973), 705–712.

14 Barton, S. *et al,* 2007, `Nutritional deficiencies in celiac disease', *Gastroenterology Clinics of North America,* Mar, 36(1), 93–108, vi.

15 Tian, L. *et al,* 2007, `Insulin resistance increases the risk of spontaneous abortion after assisted reproduction technology treatment', *Journal of Clinical Endocrinology and Metabolism,* Apr;92(4), 1430–1433. Epub 2007 Jan 23.

16 Mathias, J. *et al,* 1998, `Relation of endometriosis and neuromascular disease of the gastrointestinal tract, new insights', *Fertility and Sterility,* 70, 81–87.

17 Pritts, E. *et al,* 2001, `Fibroids and infertility: a systematic review of the evidence', *Obstetrics and Gynecology Survey,* Aug, 56(8), 483–491.

18 Casey, B., 2005, `Maternal Hypothyroidism: Maternal Fetal Outcomes', Endocrine Society Annual Meeting, May. [S7–2].

19 Moffett, A. *et al,* 2004, `Natural killer cells, miscarriage and infertility', *British Medical Journal,* 327, 1283–1285.

20 Thies, F. *et al,* 2001, `Dietary supplementation with eicosapentaenoic acid, but not with other long-chain n-3 or n-6 polyunsaturated fatty acids, decreases natural killer cell activity in healthy subjects aged >55 y', *American Journal of Clinical Nutrition,* Mar, 73(3), 539–548.

21 Makhseed, M. *et al,* 2001, `Th1 and Th2 cytokine profiles in recurrent aborters with successful pregnancy and with subsequent abortions', *Human Reproduction,* 16, 2219–2226.

22 Ng, S.C. *et al,* 2002, `Expression of intracellular Th1 normal pregnancy', *American Journal of Reproductive Immunology,* 48, 77–86.

23 Caughey, G.E. *et al,* 1996, `The effect on human tumor necrosis factor alpha and interleukin 1 beta production of diets enriched in n-3 fatty acids from vegetable oil or fish oil', *American Journal of Clinical Nutrition,* Jan, 63(1), 116–122.

24 Royal College of Obstetricians and Gynaecologists – Scientific Advisory Committee Opinion Paper 5,

Immunological testing and interventions for reproductive failure, Oct 2003.

[25] Negro, R. *et al*, 2007, `Euthyroid women with autoimmune disease undergoing assisted reproduction technologies: the role of autoimmunity and thyroid function', *Journal of Endocrinological Investigation*, 30, 1, 3–8.

[26] Gartner, R. and Gasnier, B.C., 2003, `Selenium in the treatment of autoimmune thyroiditis', *Biofactors*, 19, 3–4, 165–170.

[27] Cantorna, M.T. *et al*, 2004, `Mounting evidence for vitamin D as an environmental factor affecting autoimmune disease prevalence', *Experimental Biology and Medicine (Maywood)*, 229(11), 1136–1142.

[28] Hayes, C.E. *et al*, 2003, `The immunological functions of the vitamin D endocrine system', *Cell and Molecular Biology*, 49(2), 277–300.

[29] Panda, D.K. *et al*, 2001, `Targeted ablation of the 25-hydroxyvitamin D1 alpha-hydroxylase enzyme: evidence for skeletal, reproductive, and immune dysfunction', *Proceedings of the National Academy of Sciences of the USA*, 19, 98(13), 7498–7503.

[30] Trang, H.M. *et al*, 1998, `Evidence that vitamin D3 increases serum 25-hydroxyvitamin D more efficiently than does vitamin D', *American Journal of Clinical Nutrition*, 68, 854–858.

[31] Hoeger, G. *et al*, 2007, `Obesity and lifestyle management in polycystic ovary syndrome', *Clinical Obstetrics and Gynecology*, Mar, 50(1), 277–294.

[32] Kuller, H. *et al*, 1997, `Dietary fat and chronic diseases: epidemiologic overview', *Journal of the American Dietetic Association*, Jul, 97(7 Suppl), S9–15.

[33] Campbell, K.L. *et al*, 2007, `Effects of aerobic exercise training on estrogen metabolism in premenopausal women: a randomized controlled trial', *Cancer Epidemiology Biomarkers and Prevention*, Apr, 16(4), 731–739.

[34] Lejeune V., 2006, `Early recurrent spontaneous abortion: How to take care in 2006?', *Gynecology Obstetrique & Fertility*, Oct, 34(10), 927–937. Epub 2006 Sep 20.

STEP EIGHT ASSISTED CONCEPTION

[1] Campagne, D. *et al*, 2006, `Should fertilization treatment start with reducing stress?' *Human Reproduction*, Jul, 21(7), 1651–1658. Epub 2006 Mar 16.

[2] Sovino, H. *et al*, 2002, `Clomiphene citrate and ovulation induction', *Reproductive BioMedicine Online*, May–Jun, 4(3), 303–310.

[3] Park, S. *et al*, 2007, `Ovulatory status and follicular response predict success of clomiphene citrate-intrauterine insemination', *Fertility and Sterility*, May, 87(5), 1102–1107. Epub 2007 Jan 29.

[4] Nasseri, S. *et al*, 2001, `Clomiphene citrate in the twenty-first century', *Human Fertility (Cambridge)*, 4(3), 145–151.

[5] Haas, D.A. *et al*, 2003, `Effects of metformin on body mass index, menstrual cyclicity, and ovulation induction in women with polycystic ovary syndrome', *Fertility and Sterility*, Mar, 79(3), 469–481.

[6] Elkind, H. *et al*, 2002, `Sequential hormonal supplementation with vaginal estradiol and progesterone gel corrects the effect of clomiphene on the endometrium in oligo-ovulatory women', *Human Reproduction*, Feb, 17(2), 295–298.

[7] Karlstrom, P. *et al*, 2007, `Reducing the number of embryos transferred in Sweden-impact on delivery and multiple birth rates', *Human Reproduction*, Aug, 22(8), 2202–2207. Epub 2007 Jun 11.

[8] Bonduelle, M. et al, 2005, 'A multi-centre cohort study of the physical health of 5-year-old children conceived after intracytoplasmic sperm injection, in-vitro fertilization and natural conception', *Human Reproduction*, 20(2), 413–419.

[9] Sidani, M. *et al*, 2002, `Gynecology: select topics', *Primary Care,* Jun, 29(2), 297–321, vi.

TESTS BY POST

If you are unable to come into my clinics but are interested in some of the tests mentioned in this book, a number of them can be organised by post and the results can be sent to you with recommendations. These include the following:

Mineral analysis test This test with a hair sample checks your levels of zinc, calcium, magnesium, chromium, selenium, manganese and the heavy toxic metals – mercury, cadmium, aluminium and lead.

Vitamin D This blood test checks to see whether you have a vitamin D deficiency.

Ovarian reserve test (Plan Ahead) This blood test analyses the number of eggs remaining in your ovaries and measures your AMH, FSH and Inhibin B hormones. Your ovarian reserve for the next two years is also forecast.

Monitored cycle This test is done with saliva and the results map your female hormones over the whole cycle. Eleven samples are collected over one cycle and then posted back to the lab. This test can be useful to pick up problems with maintaining progesterone levels, luteal phase defect, early ovulation or no ovulation.

Candida test This test measures whether or not the body is producing an antibody to candida which means that there is candida overgrowth (candidiasis) through the whole body. The test is performed at home on a saliva sample and posted to the lab. The results will show whether or not you have an active candida overgrowth and it can even show whether you have had it in the past but it is not a problem now.

Leaky gut (intestinal permeability) This test evaluates whether the intestinal barrier has become permeable and unable to prevent the 'leakage' of large particles through the intestinal wall into the bloodstream. It is an easy test to do at home; you swallow a natural liquid containing different-sized molecules and then post a urine sample to the lab where they will measure if these molecules are escaping through the gut wall.

Essential fatty acid test This blood test checks for deficiencies in omega 6 and omega 3 essential fatty acids and breaks down your levels of GLA, EPA and DHA.

Gluten test This is a blood test that measures antibodies to tissue transglutaminase, a highly sensitive marker for identifying coeliac disease. If the test is positive you are reacting to gluten and removing foods containing gluten from your diet is advised.

Food allergy (intolerance) test This test measures your reaction to 233 different foods, seasonings, colourings, additives and drinks from one single blood sample.

Other tests available by post:

~ helicobacter pylori (bacteria which causes stomach ulcers)

~ stool tests to check for parasites and levels of 'good' bacteria and digestive function.

For information on any of the above please go to *www.naturalhealthpractice.com* or phone 01892 507598.

USEFUL ADDRESSES

The British Acupuncture Council
63 Jeddo Road, London W12 9HQ
Tel: 020 8735 0400
www.acupuncture.org.uk

British Infertility Counsellors Association
69 Division Street, Sheffield
South Yorkshire S4 1GE
Tel: 0114 263 1448
www.bica.net

COTS (Childlessness Overcome Through Surrogacy)
Lairg, Sutherland IV27 4EF
Tel: 01549 402777
www.surrogacy.org.uk

Daisy Network Premature Menopause Support Group
PO BOX 183, Rossendale BB4 6WZ
www.daisynetwork.org.uk

Healthy House (natural paints, water filters, etc.)
The Old Co-op, Lower Street
Ruscombe, Stroud
Gloucestershire GL6 6BU
Tel: 0845 450 5950
www.healthy-house.co.uk

Human Fertilisation and Embryology Authority (HFEA)
21 Bloomsbury Street, London WC1B 3HF
Tel: 020 7291 8200
www.hfea.gov.uk

Infertility Network (INUK)
Charter House, 43 St Leonard's Road
Bexhill-on-Sea, East Sussex TN40 IJA
Tel: 08701 188088
www.infertilitynetworkuk.com

ISSUE – The National Fertility Association
114 Lichfield Street, Walsall WS1 1SZ
Tel: 01922 722888
www.issue.co.uk

The Miscarriage Association
Clayton Hospital, Northgate
Wakefield, West Yorkshire WF1 3JS
Tel: 01924 200799
www.miscarriageassociation.org.uk

The Natural Health Practice
See page 224

Quitline (free helpline to encourage people to stop smoking)
Tel: 0800 002200

Society of Homeopaths
4a Artizan Road, Northampton NN1 4HU
Tel: 01604 621400

Verity (PCOS)
Unit AS20.01, The Aberdeen Centre
22–24 Highbury Grove
London N5 2EA
www.verity-pcos.org.uk

INDEX

The Dr Marilyn Glenville PhD Clinics
Natural Healthcare for Women

Consultations If you would like to have a consultation (either in person or by telephone), then please feel free to phone my clinic for an appointment.

I run three clinics with my team of qualified nutritionists who have all been trained by me using the integrated approach to fertility outlined in this book. The clinics are located at: Viveka in St John's Wood, London, founded by consultant gynaecologist and obstetrician Mr Yehudi Gordon; the South East Fertility Clinic in Tunbridge Wells, founded by consultant gynaecologist Mr Michael Rimington; and the third is my private clinic also in Tunbridge Wells.

To book an appointment for any of the clinic locations or for more information please contact:

The Dr Marilyn Glenville PhD Clinics
Tel: 0870 5329244 / Fax: 0870 5329255
Int. Tel: +44 1 892 515905 / Fax: +44 1 892 515914
Email: *health@marilynglenville.com*
Website: *www.marilynglenville.com*
14 St Johns Road, Tunbridge Wells, Kent TN4 9NP

Supplements and tests The Natural Health Practice (NHP) is my supplier of choice for all the supplements and tests mentioned in this book. They only carry products that I use in my clinics and are in the correct form, the right dosage levels and use the highest quality ingredients. For more information, please contact:
Website: *www.naturalhealthpractice.com*
Tel: 0845 8800915
Int. tel: +44 1 892 507598

Workshops and talks For a list of workshops and talks I will be presenting, please see my website *www.marilynglenville.com*. If you would to organise a workshop/talk near you for me to come along, call my clinic and ask for information about how to do this.

Natural news for women Each month I publish a special health digest specifically for women. It's 48 pages and packed full of useful and informative articles, breaking news stories, case studies, recipes, quick tips, questions and answers, ask Marilyn and much more. If you would like to receive a free copy or find out more information then please call 01892 507598 or email *freenaturalnews@marilynglenville.com*

Learning on the Net

Related titles of interest:

Richard Ager: *Information and Communications Technology in Primary Schools: Children or Computers in Control?* (second edition) (1-84312-042-9)

Richard Ager: *The Art of Information and Communications Technology for Teachers* (1-85346-622-0)

Alison Ball: *Help! There's a Computer in my Classroom: A Guide for Teachers* (1-84312-119-0)

Antony Smith and Simon Willcocks: *Cre8ive ICT* (1-84312-136-0)